SBA Questions for the Part 2 MRCOG

SBA Questions for the Part 2 MRCOG

The Part 2 MRCOG SBA Question Writing Group

Edited by

Amanda Jones FRCOG
Consultant Obstetrician and Gynaecologist
North Manchester General Hospital
Pennine Acute Hospitals NHS Trust
Manchester, UK

CAMBRIDGE
UNIVERSITY PRESS

CAMBRIDGE
UNIVERSITY PRESS

University Printing House, Cambridge CB2 8BS, United Kingdom

Cambridge University Press is part of the University of Cambridge.

It furthers the University's mission by disseminating knowledge in the pursuit of education, learning and research at the highest international levels of excellence.

www.cambridge.org
Information on this title: www.cambridge.org/9781107479609

© Royal College of Obstetricians & Gynaecologists 2015

This publication is in copyright. Subject to statutory exception and to the provisions of relevant collective licensing agreements, no reproduction of any part may take place without the written permission of Cambridge University Press.

First published 2015

Printed in the United Kingdom by Clays, St Ives plc

A catalogue record for this publication is available from the British Library

Library of Congress Cataloguing in Publication data
SBA Questions for the Part 2 MRCOG / the Part 2 MRCOG SBA Question Writing Group, edited by Amanda Jones.
    p. ; cm.
Includes index.
ISBN 978-1-107-47960-9
I. Jones, Amanda (Obstetrician/Gynecologist), editor.
[DNLM: 1. Gynecology – education – Great Britain – Examination Questions. 2. Obstetrics – education – Great Britain – Examination Questions. WP 18.2]
RG111
618.10076–dc23

2014044741

ISBN 978-1-107-47960-9 Paperback

Cambridge University Press has no responsibility for the persistence or accuracy of URLs for external or third-party internet websites referred to in this publication, and does not guarantee that any content on such websites is, or will remain, accurate or appropriate.

Every effort has been made in preparing this book to provide accurate and up-to-date information which is in accord with accepted standards and practice at the time of publication. Although case histories are drawn from actual cases, every effort has been made to disguise the identities of the individuals involved. Nevertheless, the authors, editors and publishers can make no warranties that the information contained herein is totally free from error, not least because clinical standards are constantly changing through research and regulation. The authors, editors and publishers therefore disclaim all liability for direct or consequential damages resulting from the use of material contained in this book. Readers are strongly advised to pay careful attention to information provided by the manufacturer of any drugs or equipment that they plan to use.

Contents

List of contributors	*page* vi
Preface	ix
INTRODUCTION	**1**
QUESTIONS	**7**
CORRECT RESPONSES	**61**
EXPLANATIONS	**65**
Index	163

Contributors

Questions written by the following members of the SBA Question Writing Group are included in this book.

DR J. ACHARYA MRCOG

DR A. AGGARWAL MRCOG

DR A. O. AHMED MRCOG

DR J. M. S. AROKIASAMY MRCOG

MISS O. J. BARNEY MRCOG

DR S. BASAK MRCOG

DR M. L. BASU MRCOG

MRS N. BHAL MRCOG

MRS R. S. BLACK MRCOG

DR H. M. CAMERON FRCOG

DR E. CHURCH MRCOG

DR E. CIANTAR MRCOG

DR K. A. J. R. COSTA MRCOG

DR J. P. DEVASEELAN MRCOG

DR F. M. FAIRLIE FRCOG

DR A. K. FORREST MRCOG

DR H. C. FRANCIS MRCOG

DR S. A. T. FRANCIS MRCOG

DR FURTADO GLEFY INACIO MRCOG

DR S. GHOSH FRCOG

DR M. GORTI MRCOG

List of contributors

DR S. GUHA MRCOG

DR P. GUPTA MRCOG

DR S. GUPTA MRCOG

DR Y. R. GURTOVAYA MRCOG

DR C. HARDIE MRCOG

DR K. JAYAPRAKASAN MRCOG

MISS A. S. JONES FRCOG

DR A. JULIANA FRCOG

DR M. KALIDINDI MRCOG

DR V. J. KAY FRCOG

DR R. A. KHAN MRCOG

DR M. KYRGIOU MRCOG

DR S. MAHADASU MRCOG

MR S. MAJUMDAR MRCOG

MR H. MARAJ MRCOG

DR R. J. MARSHALL-ROBERTS MRCOG

DR E. D. MEDD MRCOG

DR R. D. MENENI MRCOG

DR O. P. MILLING SMITH MRCOG

MR P. I. MILLS MRCOG

DR L. MOHIYIDDEEN MRCOG

DR I. A. MONTAGUE FRCOG

DR J. A. MOORE FRCOG

DR H. A. MOUSA MRCOG

MR N. A. MYERSON FRCOG

MS M. S. NAIR MRCOG

DR S. NAWAZ FRCOG

DR B. NAYAR MRCOG

DR J. C. PAGE MRCOG

DR A. S. PATIL MRCOG

DR K. I. L. PATRICK FRANZCOG

DR A. PATWARDHAN FRCOG

DR R. RAJAGOPAL MRCOG

DR K. RAMALINGAM MRCOG

DR U. RAO MRCOG

DR A. REDDY FRCOG

MISS A. E. J. REES FRCOG

List of contributors

DR A. M. SAMBROOK MRCOG

DR M. G. E. M. SAYED AHMED MRCOG

DR I. W. SCUDAMORE FRCOG

DR S. SEN MRCOG

DR S. R. SHANBHAG MRCOG

DR E. H. SHAW MRCOG

DR N. SINGH MRCOG

DR S. SIRCAR MRCOG

DR F. SOYDEMIR MRCOG

DR T. M. H. TANG MRCOG

DR T. THOMAS MRCOG

DR C. L. TOWER MRCOG

DR P. TRIPATHI MRCOG

DR A. ULLAL MRCOG

DR S. VEERAREDDY MRCOG

Preface

This book has been produced by the Royal College of Obstetricians and Gynaecologists to aid prospective candidates in their preparations for the Part 2 MRCOG examination. It reflects the work and commitment of a significant number of clinically active Fellows and Members of the College. The new SBA format required an entirely new set of peer-reviewed questions, both for the prospective examinations and for allied teaching materials. The hope is that, by studying with the aid of these questions, candidates will be able to assess their progress and enter the examination confident they are likely to achieve their goal.

The College is grateful to the individual Fellows and Members who responded to the challenge by coming together to work collectively to produce College-accredited and validated questions on contemporary clinical practice in the UK. It is an example of how the active membership of the RCOG promotes and accredits standards of care for our patients.

Mr S. M. Hughes FRCOG
Chair, Part 2 MRCOG SBA Sub-Committee

Introduction

Background
MRCOG review
A Working Party was set up in April 2012 to consider all aspects of the examination leading to Membership of the Royal College of Obstetricians and Gynaecologists (MRCOG), in order to ensure that the examination is equipped to fulfil its purpose of assessing the knowledge and certain defined skills required of specialists in women's health care. Discussions and recommendations were organized around the MRCOG's role in specialty training, the achievement of best practice regarding its format and psychometric standards, and the organizational structures required for its delivery in the present and development for the future.

The review recommended two key changes to the format of the Part 2 MRCOG, to ensure that the examination continues to strive towards the highest standards of validity and reliability:

- The introduction of a single best answer (SBA) element to replace the examination's true/false multiple choice question (MCQ) element.
- The removal of the short answer question (SAQ) element, with the existing extending matching question (EMQ) element expanded.

The new Part 2 MRCOG written examination
These changes, which take effect in March 2015, have simplified the structure of the Part 2 MRCOG written examination, with two question formats, each covered over two papers:

Previous format	New format
Paper 1: SAQs (1¾ hours)	Paper 1: 50 SBAs and 50 EMQs (3 hours)
Paper 2: 120 MCQs and 45 EMQs (2¼ hours)	Paper 2: 50 SBAs and 50 EMQs (3 hours)
Paper 3: 120 MCQs and 45 EMQs (2¼ hours)	

In each of the two new papers, the SBA element contributes 40% of the total marks and the EMQ element contributes 60% of the total marks. The higher tariff for EMQs reflects the increased amount of time required to answer each EMQ when compared with each SBA.

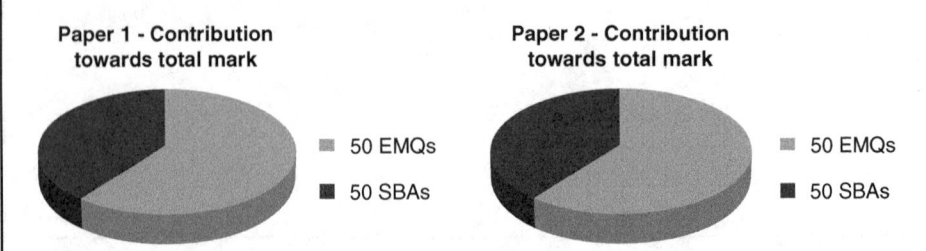

Paper 1 - Contribution towards total mark
- 50 EMQs
- 50 SBAs

Paper 2 - Contribution towards total mark
- 50 EMQs
- 50 SBAs

The introduction of SBAs in the Part 2 MRCOG follows the successful introduction of SBAs in the Part 1 MRCOG in 2012, in part at the expense of the contribution of that examination's MCQ element, with the latter format increasingly viewed as insufficiently robust for high-stakes examinations. Indeed, because of its promotion of factual regurgitation over higher-order thinking, lack of professional authenticity, and the encouragement of cue-seeking behaviours such as question spotting and exhaustive practice, the MCQ format is perceived as less fair and less rigorous than other question formats.

The replacement of MCQs with an expanded SBA element addresses these shortcomings without undermining either the breadth of knowledge covered in the examination or the reliability with which this is assessed. Indeed, the greater discrimination between good and bad candidates that individual SBA questions offer compared with MCQs ensures that the reliability of the Part 2 MRCOG should improve. These two aims – a greater breadth of knowledge tested more effectively and a greater reliability – are further achieved by the removal of the SAQ element from the Part 2 MRCOG, which is the logical conclusion of a process that has seen its contribution to the overall score diminish over the past 10 years as more effective assessment techniques have been developed. Assessment is often the driving force behind learning, and the change in format allows the questions to be more relevant to clinical practice and thus a more valid assessment.

Blueprinting

'Blueprinting' refers to the process of mapping the examination to the syllabus to ensure sufficient coverage of all domains and modules. A Part 2 MRCOG written examination composed only of best answer question formats (SBA and EMQ) reflects progress in assessment methodology. However, it does pose a question regarding the division of labour between two question formats that, in essence, share a number of similarities. In fact, the way in which EMQs within the Part 2 MRCOG have evolved to include detailed clinical information, requiring an effective synthesis of this as well as subsequent application of knowledge, ensures that they have become equipped to perform a different function from that designed for SBAs within the Part 2 MRCOG.

For this reason, SBAs and EMQs can coexist comfortably within the Part 2 MRCOG, and careful consideration has been given to how each question format will contribute to assessing the material of the examination's syllabus, with questions generated to identify areas of best fit. The blueprinting approach will accommodate the fact that domains such as aetiology, basic sciences, epidemiology, natural history and statistics/audit lend themselves to assessment by SBAs. Meanwhile, investigations, diagnosis and management are tested more effectively using EMQs. Such a distribution of topics is, however, designed to be a guide rather than unnecessarily prescriptive.

The MRCOG syllabus underpins the blueprint grid and the grid ensures that the breadth of the syllabus is covered in each exam.

Standard setting

A significant benefit of the introduction, in SBAs, of a question format similar in nature to existing EMQs is that the new Part 2 MRCOG format can accommodate an extension of a successful approach to standard setting in this element of the examination. The Angoff method[1] has proven to be an effective method of identifying the minimum standard for the Part 2 MRCOG's optically marked elements and will continue to be used for the SBA paper.

Summary

The move from true/false MCQs, which rely on rote learning, and SAQs, which are difficult to mark consistently, will increase the validity and reliability of the MRCOG exam. All questions are reviewed by teams of consultants prior to inclusion in the bank of questions for the exam and are edited to ensure they are not ambiguous and are relevant to the standard of an ST5 trainee. The questions are reviewed on a regular basis to ensure that they are up to date and reflect current clinical practice in the UK. The pass mark varies for each exam depending on the difficulty of the questions. This is set prior to each exam using the Angoff method – assessing the proportion of borderline candidates who would be expected to get the right answer to the question. All questions used in the examination are reviewed to assess their ability to discriminate between good and poor candidates. Any question with poor or negative discrimination may be rewritten or discarded.

Modern examinations need to assess clinical knowledge and ability. By moving to SBA and EMQ styles of questions, the MRCOG exam goes beyond basic knowledge and allows assessment of clinical reasoning and data interpretation. This reflects the doctor's clinical practice more accurately. With 200 questions in the two papers, reliability is ensured.

The SBA Regional Question Writing Model

Adapted from an article first published in O&G, the RCOG membership magazine

Members of the RCOG regularly ask how they can become more fully involved with the work of the College. In March 2013, Council accepted the recommendation of the MRCOG Review Working Party that the Part 2 MRCOG examination should replace its multiple choice questions (MCQs) and short answer questions (SAQs) with single best answer questions (SBAs). By December 2013, 93 consultants from all over the British Isles had volunteered to undertake the crucial work of building the College's bank of new SBAs, working in 16 regional question-writing groups. For many of these consultants, this has been their first substantive involvement with the work of the College post-CCT.

In February 2013, Mr Kevin Hayes MRCOG, the Chair of the College's Assessment Sub-Committee, ran a workshop on the writing of SBAs for the existing and new members of the MCQ Sub-Committee, which was now reconstituted as the

---

[1] The Angoff method is a widely used criterion-referenced approach whereby examiners are required to consider the notion of a 'borderline' candidate (i.e. a hypothetical minimally competent candidate) and rate questions by considering how difficult they would be for this borderline candidate. The results of this exercise are then used to inform the pass mark.

SBA Sub-Committee. This event was followed in March by a workshop for all 93 of the new regional question writers.

After the workshop, all members were asked to write four questions each for review in the May Sub-Committee meeting, and this resulted in the submission of a very respectable total of 240. By the end of summer 2014, over 500 questions had been produced and reviewed by the SBA Sub-Committee, some of which have been used in this publication.

The concept of regional question writing groups fits very well with the College's policy of the regionalization of College activity to make it less London-centric. It has proved to be an efficient and enjoyable means of building up an entirely new bank of questions to ensure that the MRCOG retains its primacy as a world-class examination.

Single best answer (SBA) questions

What is an SBA?

Single best answer questions – also referred to as 'best of five' questions – usually consist of a stem describing a scenario, a lead-in question, and five plausible options labelled a–e, one of which is clearly the most appropriate. They are designed to assess application of knowledge and clinical reasoning.

Although the five options are plausible – some may even be partially correct – there is always one answer that is clearly the best.

A typical SBA is shown below:

A 24-year-old presents at 27 weeks into her second pregnancy feeling unwell, with backache, fever and rigors. She has a temperature of 39.5 °C. Urinalysis shows leucocytes and protein +++. Her blood pressure is 80/50.

Which is the most appropriate action to take?

a) Admit to ICU/HDU for intravenous antibiotics and supportive care
b) Arrange ultrasound of renal tract
c) Commence 7-day course of oral antibiotics
d) Give intramuscular steroids to promote fetal lung maturity
e) Make referral for physicians to review

Answering the questions

For each Part 2 MRCOG examination paper, the SBA answer sheet is numbered 1–50. Against each number there are five lozenges labelled a–e:

1 [a] [b] [c] [d] [e]

2 [a] [b] [c] [d] [e]

3 [a] [b] [c] [d] [e]

4 [a] [b] [c] [d] [e]

5 [a] [b] [c] [d] [e]

Answer each question by boldly blacking out the letter that corresponds to the single best answer in the options list:

1	■	[b]	[c]	[d]	[e]
2	[a]	■	[c]	[d]	[e]
3	■	[b]	[c]	[d]	[e]
4	[a]	[b]	■	[d]	[e]
5	[a]	[b]	[c]	■	[e]

Candidates may mark their responses in the question book and then transfer them to the answer sheet, but be aware that this will take longer and all answers must be transferred fully within the time allowed for the examination.

The 200 SBA questions included in this book have all been produced by the Part 2 SBA Regional Question Writing Group and reviewed by the Part 2 MRCOG SBA Sub-Committee, following the same process and meeting the same standards as the questions that will be used in the actual examination. The questions used in this book will not appear in the examination.

Questions

Questions

1

A 32-year-old woman attends her general practitioner surgery concerned that she has forgotten to take her oral contraceptive pills for the previous two days, having taken the first five tablets in the packet. She had unprotected sexual intercourse last night.

What is the most appropriate contraceptive advice?

a) Advise her to miss her forgotten pills and take her next pill at the usual time
b) Advise her that you recommend emergency contraception
c) Advise her to take her forgotten pills now and the next one at the usual time
d) Advise her to take her forgotten pills now and the next one at the usual time and start the next packet omitting the pill-free 7 days
e) Advise her to take her forgotten pills now and the next one at the usual time and use additional contraceptive for the next 7 days

2

A community midwife booking a woman at 10 weeks of gestation is concerned that she might have had female genital mutilation (FGM). She speaks to the registrar, who enquires about the patient's country of origin.

Which country has the highest reported prevalence of FGM?

a) Nigeria
b) Somalia
c) Togo
d) Tanzania
e) Yemen

3

A 33-year-old woman has primary infertility due to bilateral hydrosalpinges. She has been referred for assisted reproduction. She is otherwise fit and well with no significant past medical history of note.

What initial treatment would optimize her chances of pregnancy with in-vitro fertilization (IVF)?

a) Aspiration of hydrosalpinx fluid
b) Hysteroscopic proximal tubal occlusion

c) Laparoscopic proximal tubal occlusion
d) Salpingectomy
e) Salpingostomy

4

A 30-year-old woman had a vaginal delivery and also required manual removal of the placenta under spinal anaesthesia. She is known to be rhesus negative and her baby is confirmed to be rhesus positive. The Kleihauer test shows fetomaternal haemorrhage (FMH) of 5 mL.

How much anti-D should this woman receive?

a) 500 IU
b) 625 IU
c) 750 IU
d) 875 IU
e) 1000 IU

5

You are a working as a fifth-year specialist trainee. A first-year specialist trainee asks you to observe her taking a history and performing an abdominal examination.

Which assessment tool is most appropriate to provide feedback on her history-taking skills?

a) CbD (case-based discussion)
b) Mini-CEX (mini clinical evaluation exercise)
c) OSATS (objective structured assessment of technical skill)
d) PQ (patient questionnaire)
e) TO1 (team observation)

6

You have performed a hysterectomy on a 40-year-old woman for heavy menstrual bleeding. She has no significant medical history. Histology shows completely excised cervical intraepithelial neoplasia (CIN) grade 3. She is on routine recall for her smears and they have all been normal previously.

According to the NHS Cervical Screening Programme (NHSCSP) guidelines, when should she have vaginal vault cytology?

a) 3 and 6 months
b) 6 and 12 months
c) 6 and 18 months
d) 6, 12 and 18 months
e) 6, 12 and 24 months

7

A couple, both aged 28, have been trying to conceive for over two years. They are both fit and well, with a normal body mass index (BMI), and are non-smokers. Following thorough investigation, they have been given a diagnosis of unexplained subfertility.

What treatment would NICE (the National Institute for Health and Care Excellence) recommend is offered to this couple?

a) Clomifene citrate
b) Intracytoplasmic sperm injection (ICSI)

c) Intrauterine insemination (IUI)
d) In-vitro fertilization (IVF)
e) Letrozole

8

A 41-year-old primigravida with a body mass index (BMI) of 31 attends the antenatal clinic at 10 weeks of gestation. Her father has type 2 diabetes. In this pregnancy, she will require aspirin 75 mg daily and will require screening for gestational diabetes with a glucose tolerance test (GTT).

At what gestation should she commence the aspirin and be screened for diabetes?

a) Aspirin from 12 weeks and GTT between 16 and 20 weeks
b) Aspirin from 12 weeks and GTT between 24 and 28 weeks
c) Aspirin from 16 weeks and GTT between 16 and 20 weeks
d) Aspirin from 16 weeks and GTT between 24 and 28 weeks
e) Aspirin from 16 weeks and GTT between 28 and 32 weeks

9

A 35-year-old woman who has had two previous vaginal deliveries at 40 weeks has tested positive for HIV on antenatal screening. At booking, her viral load is reported as 150 copies/mL. She is otherwise well and is commenced on HAART (highly active antiretroviral therapy). At 36 weeks, her viral load is 75 copies/mL and there are no other obstetric complications.

What is the most appropriate delivery plan?

a) Await spontaneous labour
b) Caesarean section at 38 weeks
c) Caesarean section at 39 weeks
d) Induction of labour at 37 weeks
e) Induction of labour after 41 weeks

10

A 38-year-old primiparous woman attends for review following her 20-week scan. She has a history of systemic lupus erythematosus (SLE) diagnosed five years ago, predominantly causing joint and skin symptoms. On scan, the baby's heart was structurally normal with a rate of 80 bpm.

What is the most likely cause of the fetal heart rate of 80 bpm?

a) Anticardiolipin antibodies
b) Anti-double-stranded DNA
c) Anti-nuclear antibodies
d) Ribonuclear protein antibodies
e) Sjögren's syndrome A antibodies

11

A 46-year-old woman had total abdominal hysterectomy for heavy menstrual bleeding due to a multiple fibroid uterus. Postoperatively, she had extreme difficulty in climbing the stairs. There is also some paraesthesia over the anterior and medial thigh as well as the medial aspect of the calf.

Which nerve has been injured during the operation?

a) Femoral nerve
b) Genitofemoral nerve
c) Ilioinguinal nerve
d) Obturator nerve
e) Sciatic nerve

12

A 21-year-old woman presents four days after unprotected sexual intercourse requesting emergency contraception. She is undergoing treatment for *Chlamydia*.

What is the most appropriate medication?

a) Levonorgestrel
b) Medroxyprogesterone acetate
c) Mifepristone
d) Norethisterone acetate
e) Ulipristal acetate

13

A woman attends the antenatal clinic at 12 weeks of gestation requesting cervical cerclage as she has previously had a LLETZ (large loop excision of the transformation zone) for cervical dyskaryosis and is anxious she will deliver prematurely.

Under what circumstance would cervical cerclage be indicated?

a) At 20 weeks she has a cervical length of 23 mm on transvaginal ultrasound scan
b) She had a previous delivery at 33 weeks
c) She has previously had a miscarriage at 18 weeks of gestation
d) The pregnancy is a twin pregnancy
e) There is funnelling on transvaginal ultrasound scan at 23 weeks

14

A woman with a body mass index (BMI) of 63 has a complicated labour and delivery and nearly dies.

Which of the following causes of maternal mortality is independent of her BMI?

a) Amniotic fluid embolism
b) Anaesthetic complications
c) Pre-eclampsia
d) Sepsis
e) Venous thromboembolism

15

You review a woman who is currently 30 weeks pregnant in her second pregnancy. She had deep venous thrombosis (DVT) in her last pregnancy. In her current pregnancy, she was commenced on prophylactic low-molecular-weight heparin (LMWH) once a day.

Compared to unfractionated heparin, which of the following statements about LMWH is most accurate?

a) LMWH binds more effectively to antithrombin III and enhances the inhibition of coagulation factor IXa
b) LMWH binds more strongly to endothelial cells and platelets

c) LMWH has a higher bioavailability at lower dose when administered subcutaneously
d) LMWH has a similar effect on bones and can induce osteoporosis
e) LMWH has a similar half life

16

A general practitioner has referred a 36-year-old woman to gynaecology outpatients because of her symptoms of intermenstrual bleeding as well as subfertility. Her pelvic scan is as follows:

Anteverted uterus measures 77 × 50 × 42 mm.
Myometrial appearances are suggestive of adenomyosis.
Endometrial thickness is 7 mm with a 10 × 15 mm mass at the fundus: ?polyp.
Both ovaries appear normal, with a 13 mm follicle in the left ovary.
No free fluid or adnexal masses seen.
She enquires about other investigations to confirm the presence of an endometrial polyp.

Which of the following modalities is considered to be the gold standard for diagnosing endometrial polyps?

a) CT scan of pelvis
b) Hysteroscopy
c) Pelvic ultrasound
d) Saline infusion sonogram
e) Transvaginal ultrasound

17

A 46-year-old woman presents for assessment prior to a planned admission for abdominal hysterectomy. She has well-controlled type 2 diabetes and her body mass index (BMI) is 42. Her mother had a pulmonary embolism after hip replacement, but she was investigated and found to be negative for thrombophilia. The indication for hysterectomy is menorrhagia and anaemia caused by a large fibroid uterus. Her preoperative haemoglobin is 122 g/L.

What is the most important factor influencing a plan for anticoagulant prophylaxis?

a) Her age
b) Her BMI
c) Her family history of thrombosis
d) Her fibroid uterus
e) Her history of anaemia

18

A 25-year-old para 1 woman sustained a 3a perineal tear following an instrumental delivery. She attends her postnatal follow-up appointment. She has no faecal incontinence, has no incontinence of flatus and the perineum has healed well.

What advice would you offer this woman with regard to subsequent delivery?

a) Avoiding prolonged second stage eliminates the risk of a third-degree tear
b) Early epidural reduces the risk of a third-degree tear
c) Elective caesarean section eliminates the risk of faecal incontinence in later life
d) Prophylactic episiotomy reduces the risk of a third-degree tear
e) Subsequent vaginal delivery is associated with a small additional risk of developing faecal incontinence

19

A 32-year-old woman is brought into the emergency department with a one-day history of fever, rigors, abdominal pain and heavy lochia. She had an uncomplicated spontaneous vaginal delivery two days ago. On arrival, she has a temperature of 39 °C, a heart rate of 143 bpm, a blood pressure of 82/50 mmHg and a respiratory rate of 40/min.

Following initial resuscitation, what is the most appropriate immediate management?

a) Blood cultures and vaginal swabs
b) Broad-spectrum IV antibiotics
c) Evacuation of retained products of conception
d) IV dopamine
e) IV immunoglobulin

20

A 45-year-old woman underwent a total abdominal hysterectomy for heavy menstrual bleeding. In the postoperative period she develops weakness of hip flexion and adduction and is unable to extend the knee. On examination the knee jerk reflex is lost and there is altered sensation over the medial aspect of thigh and calf.

What nerve is most likely to have been damaged?

a) Femoral nerve
b) Genitofemoral nerve
c) Ilioinguinal nerve
d) Obturator nerve
e) Pudendal nerve

21

A primigravid woman attends the antenatal clinic with a query. She is a teacher and is 16 weeks pregnant and has been exposed to a student with slapped cheek syndrome about four weeks ago. As far as she is aware, she has never had this herself and is concerned about her pregnancy. A blood test is negative for IgG and positive for maternal IgM antibodies for parvovirus. An ultrasound scan reveals a normal viable pregnancy.

What advice would you give this woman regarding follow-up?

a) She can be reassured and discharged if a second scan in 4 weeks' time is normal
b) She can be reassured and discharged in view of the normal scan
c) She should have 4-weekly growth scans from 28 weeks
d) She should have fortnightly ultrasound scans until 30 weeks. If the scans are normal she can be reassured and discharged
e) She should have fortnightly ultrasound scans until delivery

22

Following the effective management of a shoulder dystocia, a first-year trainee approaches you to learn how to perform the manoeuvres to manage shoulder dystocia.

What is the most effective way of achieving this learning?

a) Attending a lecture
b) Brainstorming
c) Case-based discussion
d) Electronic learning
e) Simulation training

23

A primiparous woman presents two days after a normal vaginal delivery complaining of feeling unwell. On examination, she has a temperature of 38 °C, pulse rate of 110 bpm and blood pressure of 90/50 mmHg. There are no localizing signs of infection. Blood tests are performed.

What test result would indicate a severe sepsis?

a) C-reactive protein 53 mg/L (normal < 10)
b) Plasma glucose 12.2 mmol/L (normal 3.6–6.1)
c) Serum creatinine 90 mmol/L (normal 53–97)
d) Serum lactate 5 mmol/L (normal 0.5–2.2)
e) White cell count 13.1×10^9/L (normal $4–11 \times 10^9$)

24

A 59-year-old para 2 woman presents with postmenopausal bleeding. She is found to have an endometrial thickness of 11 mm on ultrasound scan and is booked for an outpatient hysteroscopy.

What is the ideal size of hysteroscope for her procedure?

a) 2.2 mm hysteroscope with 2.5–3 mm sheath
b) 2.7 mm hysteroscope with 3–3.5 mm sheath
c) 2.7 mm hysteroscope with 4–5 mm sheath
d) 3 mm hysteroscope with 3.5–4 mm sheath
e) 3 mm hysteroscope with 4.5–5 mm sheath

25

A 25-year-old woman has been having persistently high blood pressure of > 150/100 mmHg for three days following delivery with no biochemical or haematological abnormalities. She has no underlying medical problems and was not on any antihypertensive drugs during the pregnancy. She is breastfeeding.

Which is the most appropriate antihypertensive agent that can be prescribed for her?

a) Amlodipine
b) Bendroflumethiazide
c) Candesartan
d) Enalapril
e) Methyldopa

26

In the Confidential Enquiry into Maternal Deaths, sepsis was the leading cause of maternal mortality in the UK between 2006 and 2008.

Which one of the following most accurately represents the mortality rate of severe sepsis with acute organ dysfunction?

a) 1–10%
b) 21–30%
c) 41–50%
d) 61–70%
e) 81–90%

27

You are about to repair a second-degree tear under local anaesthetic in a woman with no previous analgesia. Her most recent weight in pregnancy was 50 kg.

What is the maximum volume of 1% lidocaine (when not mixed with adrenaline) that can be used?

a) 10 mL
b) 15 mL
c) 20 mL
d) 25 mL
e) 30 mL

28

An ST6 doctor (postgraduate doctor in year 6 of specialty training) attends an appraisal meeting with her educational supervisor.

Which one of the following statements best describes the appraisal process?

a) Personal and educational development are discussed with agreed goals
b) The educational supervisor provides an assessment and review of performance
c) The educational supervisor provides the trainee with objective evidence of her progress
d) The educational supervisor reviews progress and recommends the educational targets to be achieved
e) This is a summative assessment of the trainee's progress

29

A medical student is interested in learning about enhanced recovery in gynaecology.

Which of the following principles is *not* part of an enhanced recovery pathway?

a) Antibiotic prophylaxis following the skin incision
b) Avoidance of intraoperative hypothermia
c) Complex carbohydrate drinks 4 hours prior to surgery
d) Early postoperative feeding
e) Verbal and written information for the patient explaining the perioperative pathway

30

You have just completed the last case on the afternoon theatre list, having assisted with a hysterectomy with your consultant, and she requests you to complete the WHO sign-out while she finishes writing up the operating notes.

Which of the following is *not* usually part of a WHO surgical sign-out?

a) Has it been confirmed that instruments, swabs and sharps counts are complete?
b) Has the name of the procedure been recorded?
c) Has the scheduling of the list workload been appropriate?
d) Have any equipment problems been identified that need to be addressed?
e) Have the specimens been labelled (including patient name)?

31

The cardiovascular system undergoes immense physiological changes in pregnancy.

Which of the following parameters does *not* change in pregnancy?

a) Cardiac output
b) Central venous pressure
c) Heart rate
d) Stroke volume
e) Systemic vascular resistance

32

There are huge changes in the coagulation system in pregnancy.

Which of the following components of the coagulation system does *not* change in an uncomplicated pregnancy?

a) Factor IX
b) Fibrinogen
c) Platelets
d) Protein S
e) Von Willebrand's factor

33

In the most recent Confidential Enquiry into Maternal Deaths (2006–08), sepsis was the leading cause of direct maternal deaths.

Among the direct maternal deaths due to sepsis, which were the most common risk factors to predict those who died?

a) Body mass index (BMI) 40+, over 40 years, primiparity
b) BMI 40+, under 40 years, multiparity
c) BMI 40+, under 40 years, primiparity
d) Normal BMI, under 40 years, primiparity
e) Normal BMI, under 40 years, multiparity

34

A 23-year-old primigravid woman presents at the emergency department at six weeks of gestation with threatened miscarriage. On examination, her vital signs are normal and abdomen is soft and there is minimal tenderness on deep palpation. On speculum examination, there is a small amount of brown (old) blood in the vagina. A transvaginal ultrasound scan shows an intrauterine gestation sac, measuring 38 × 25 × 20 mm. A yolk sac is visible, and a fetal pole is visible measuring 6 mm. No fetal heart activity is seen. A small area of subchorionic haemorrhage is seen.

What would be the best management plan for her?

a) Arrange for a dating scan at 12 weeks
b) Arrange for a repeat scan after 7 days
c) Arrange for a serial serum beta-hCG level
d) Arrange for a serum progesterone level
e) Arrange surgical management of miscarriage

35

A 35-year-old primigravida is referred to the antenatal clinic at 32 weeks of gestation. The midwife performed a blood test to check her liver function tests a week ago when she had an itchy rash. The rash has disappeared and she is no longer itchy. Her blood pressure is 110/70 mmHg and there is no proteinuria. Examination is normal. The results show:

Total bilirubin 7 μmol/L (normal 0–17)
Alkaline phosphatase 183 IU/L (normal 30–130)
Alanine transaminase 28 IU/L (normal 0–40)
Albumin 32 g/L (normal 35–46)

What is the most appropriate blood test?

a) Check prothrombin time
b) Check serum total bile acids
c) No blood test required
d) Repeat liver function tests
e) Test for viral hepatitis

36

A 28-year-old nulliparous woman has had two consecutive miscarriages in the first trimester. She is referred with a further non-viable pregnancy at eight weeks of gestation.

What is the most appropriate genetic test to perform?

a) Karyotype both partners
b) Karyotype chorionic villus sample in next pregnancy
c) Karyotype father
d) Karyotype mother
e) Karyotype products of conception

37

A nulliparous woman presents with lower abdominal pain in early pregnancy. The human chorionic gonadotrophin (hCG) level is 986 IU/L. At laparoscopy the following is found:

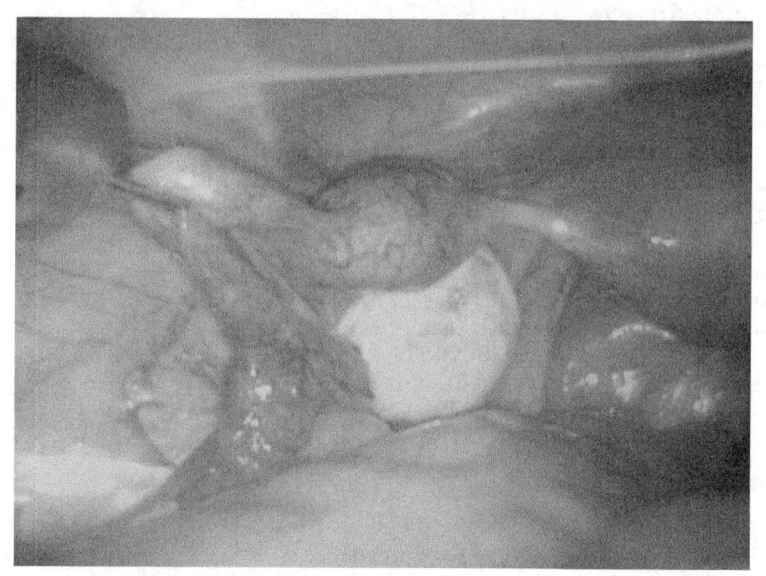

There is no other abnormality seen in the pelvis.
What is the most appropriate management option?

a) Inject methotrexate into mass
b) Intramuscular methotrexate injection
c) Left salpingectomy
d) Left salpingo-oophorectomy
e) Left salpingostomy

38

A 34-year-old primigravida presents to the maternity assessment unit with a second episode of decreased fetal movements at 38 + 4 weeks of gestation. She is known to be low risk and has had an otherwise uneventful pregnancy. An ultrasound scan a week ago was normal, with the baby on the 50th centile.

What is the most appropriate management option?

a) Advise formal kick counting and review in 2 days
b) Arrange a biophysical profile and, if normal, reassure
c) Consider induction of labour
d) Perform cardiotocography (CTG) and arrange a further scan
e) Perform a CTG and, if normal, reassure

39

A 52-year-old woman has recently been diagnosed with cervical intraepithelial neoplasia grade 3 (CIN3) following severe dyskaryosis on a cervical smear. A LLETZ specimen shows CIN3 incompletely excised at the endocervical margin.

What is the most appropriate next step in her management?

a) Colposcopy and smear in 6 months
b) Loop excision immediately
c) Loop excision in 6 months

d) Smear in 6 months
e) Smear and high-risk human papillomavirus (HR-HPV) DNA testing in 6 months

40

A 32-year-old woman with dull lower abdominal pain and bloating had a pelvic ultrasound scan arranged by her general practitioner. The results show a simple 30 mm right-sided ovarian cyst. There are no other concerns.

What is the most appropriate next step in her management?

a) Arrange for a repeat scan in 4 months
b) Arrange for a repeat scan in a year
c) Arrange further imaging with MRI/CT
d) Check serum CA-125
e) Reassure and discharge without follow-up

41

A 34-year-old primigravid woman attends for her booking scan at 12 weeks of gestation. The report shows a live twin pregnancy with T sign present on ultrasound scan. The crown–rump length is equivalent to 12 + 5 for both twins.

What would you document in her plan of care?

a) Aim for delivery at 36–37 weeks
b) Caesarean section is the recommended mode of delivery
c) Quad test screening at 16 weeks
d) Refer to fetal medicine unit
e) Serial scan every 4 weeks

42

A 37-year-old woman is due to have a diagnostic laparoscopy to investigate chronic pelvic pain. The overall risk of serious complications is 1 in 500.

What is the most appropriate way to explain this risk verbally?

a) Common
b) Rare
c) Unusual
d) Uncommon
e) Very rare

43

A 54-year-old woman was referred to the outpatient hysteroscopy clinic with a history of a single episode of vaginal bleeding, which lasted for a day. She had her last period two years ago. A transvaginal ultrasound scan showed an endometrial thickness of 6 mm. She is nulliparous and her body mass index (BMI) is 47. She is very anxious and is requesting pain relief.

What is the most appropriate option for pain relief?

a) Codeine tablets orally about an hour before the procedure
b) Conscious sedation
c) Infiltration of local anaesthetic into the cervix
d) Instillation of local anaesthetic into the cervical canal
e) Not suitable for outpatient procedure; list under general anaesthesia

44

A woman who is 12 weeks pregnant has a first-trimester screening for Down's syndrome, which shows a high-risk result. The woman undergoes amniocentesis at 15 weeks of gestation.

What is the additional risk of miscarriage following amniocentesis?

a) 0.5%
b) 1%
c) 2%
d) 2.5%
e) 3%

45

You are performing a diagnostic laparoscopy on a 28-year-old woman with a body mass index (BMI) of 25 who has not had any previous surgery. You have introduced the Veress needle safely and started gas insufflations.

What intra-abdominal pressure should be achieved to safely insert the primary trocar?

a) 5–10 mmHg
b) 10–15 mmHg
c) 15–20 mmHg
d) 20–25 mmHg
e) 25–30 mmHg

46

You have performed a hysteroscopy to investigate postmenopausal bleeding with a 5 mm hysteroscope, and while performing the curettage you suspect a uterine perforation.

What is the most appropriate management plan?

a) Administration of antibiotics and observation
b) Hysteroscopic repair
c) Laparoscopy
d) Laparotomy
e) Urgent postoperative imaging

47

A 35-year-old para 2 woman is referred to the gynaecology department with a history of worsening frequency, urgency and urge incontinence. There is no history of stress urinary incontinence, recurrent urinary tract infections, haematuria or prolapse symptoms. Urinalysis is normal.

Following a detailed history and examination, what would be the next most appropriate method of assessment?

a) Filling and voiding cystometry
b) Flexible cystoscopy
c) Renal tract ultrasound scan
d) Three-day bladder diary
e) Urine cytology

48

A 30-year-old woman is delivered at 27 weeks of gestation due to severe pre-eclampsia.

What is the risk of recurrence of severe pre-eclampsia in the subsequent pregnancy?

a) 20–25%
b) 30–35%
c) 40–45%
d) 50–55%
e) 60–65%

49

A 45-year-old woman with symptomatic fibroids is considering uterine artery embolization (UAE). She has read that her symptoms might return after the procedure.

She should be informed that the risk of requiring further treatment for recurrent symptoms by five years is:

a) 5%
b) 10%
c) 15%
d) 20%
e) 25%

50

A primigravida was delivered by Neville Barnes forceps for a pathological cardiotocogram (CTG). Following delivery, a 3b perineal tear was diagnosed.

What is a 3b injury?

a) Both external and internal anal sphincters and anal epithelium torn
b) Both external and internal anal sphincters torn
c) Less than 50% of external anal sphincter thickness torn
d) More than 50% of external anal sphincter thickness torn
e) Perineal muscles torn

51

A 26-year-old woman has recently been diagnosed as being HIV positive. Her general practitioner notices that her first smear last year was negative, and contacts you for advice about the frequency of cervical smears for this woman.

How often should her cervical smears be undertaken?

a) Every 6 months
b) Every 6 months for 2 years and then routine recall
c) Annually
d) Every 3 years
e) Every 5 years

52

A 34-year-old woman is diagnosed to have vulval intraepithelial neoplasia grade 3 (VIN3) on a punch biopsy from a vulval lesion.

What is the recommended treatment for this condition?

a) Interferon therapy
b) Laser ablation of the lesion
c) Local surgical excision
d) Simple vulvectomy
e) Topical imiquimod cream

53

A woman with a history of depression attends for pre-pregnancy counselling. She asks about antidepressant use in pregnancy.

Which is the antidepressant with the lowest known risk in pregnancy?

a) Amitriptyline
b) Fluoxetine
c) Nortriptyline
d) Paroxetine
e) Venlafaxine

54

A 56-year-old woman has been diagnosed with an overactive bladder (OAB).

What is the first line of treatment for this woman?

a) Bladder training for 6 weeks
b) Botulinum toxin injection into the bladder
c) OAB drug regime and bladder training
d) Percutaneous posterior tibial nerve stimulation
e) Transcutaneous sacral nerve stimulation

55

A 37-year-old woman is seen in clinic after her third consecutive early pregnancy loss (miscarriage).

What is the most likely cause of recurrent miscarriage?

a) Antiphospholipid syndrome
b) Cervical factors
c) Genetic causes
d) Genital infections
e) Uterine anatomical abnormality

56

A community midwife asks for advice regarding a 20 weeks pregnant woman whose son has developed chickenpox a day before. The woman is not sure if she has had chickenpox herself. She is otherwise well.

What will be the most appropriate immediate management?

a) Ask her to come back if she develops any rash
b) Check varicella-zoster virus immunity and wait for result
c) Give varicella-zoster immunoglobulin as soon as possible
d) Reassure and do nothing, as she is completely asymptomatic
e) Treat with oral aciclovir for 7 days

57

A 26-year-old primigravid woman attends the antenatal clinic at 12 weeks of gestation in view of a family history of a bleeding disorder. She too gives a history of a significant bleeding tendency, including spontaneous joint bleeds. A von Willebrand profile is performed and she is found to have unmeasurable von Willebrand factor (vWF) levels and severely low factor VIII (FVIII) levels.

What is the most likely diagnosis?

a) Haemophilia A
b) Haemophilia B
c) Type I von Willebrand's disease
d) Type 2a von Willebrand's disease
e) Type 3 von Willebrand's disease

58

You are writing a guideline about prevention of venous thromboembolism (VTE) in pregnancy and you need to include information on background epidemiology.

What is the overall incidence of VTE in pregnancy and the puerperium?

a) 0.1–0.2/1000
b) 1–2/1000
c) 5–10/1000
d) 20–40/1000
e) 60–80/1000

59

A 34-year-old woman in her second pregnancy is seen in the antenatal clinic at 12 weeks. Three years ago she had a placental abruption resulting in a preterm delivery at 26 weeks. She has no other relevant history.

What is her risk of another abruption in this pregnancy?

a) 2–3%
b) 4–5%
c) 6–7%
d) 9–10%
e) 11–12%

60

A 19-year-old primigravida presents to the delivery suite in early labour. Her pregnancy has been low risk throughout. She is concerned about her delivery and would be very reluctant to consent to an operative vaginal delivery if she needed one.

Which of the following is most likely to increase her chances of achieving a spontaneous vaginal delivery?

a) Commencing pushing as soon as she is fully dilated
b) Continuous support in labour
c) Documenting progress on a partogram
d) Lying in the supine position during labour
e) Use of epidural for analgesia in labour

61

A 28-year-old woman in her first pregnancy attends the antenatal clinic at eight weeks because of a strong family history of thromboembolism. Her general practitioner has performed a thrombophilia screen, which is reported as abnormal.

Which statement concerning the results of thrombophilia screening during pregnancy is correct?

a) Antithrombin levels are decreased
b) Factor V Leiden mutation cannot be diagnosed
c) Protein C levels are decreased
d) Protein S levels are decreased
e) Prothrombin gene mutation cannot be diagnosed

62

A woman with a history of depression is referred for pre-conception counselling. She is concerned about her risk of postpartum psychosis.

From the following list, what is her risk of developing postpartum psychosis?

a) 2 per 1000
b) 3 per 1000
c) 4 per 1000
d) 5 per 1000
e) 6 per 1000

63

The Confidential Enquiries into UK maternal deaths cover deaths directly and indirectly related to pregnancy.

The eighth report (2006–08) reported that the most common cause of indirect maternal death was:

a) Cardiac disease
b) Epilepsy
c) Hypertensive disease
d) Sepsis
e) Thromboembolism

64

A 40-year-old woman underwent a LLETZ (large loop excision of the transformation zone) procedure in a hospital in England and the histology report showed incomplete excision of cervical intraepithelial neoplasia grade 3 (CIN3). Follow-up smear and human papillomavirus (HPV) testing at six months are negative.

What is the correct follow-up for this woman?

a) Annual smear for 10 years
b) Smear and HPV testing at 6 months
c) Smear and HPV testing at 12 months
d) Smear and HPV testing at 3 years
e) Smear and HPV testing at 5 years

65

You are called to obstetric theatre to see a woman who has a retained placenta. On examining her, you recognize that in addition to the retained placenta she has a partial uterine inversion. Your initial attempt to manually reduce the inversion is not successful.

What can the anaesthetist administer to assist you in reducing the inversion?

a) Carboprost 125 µg IV
b) Ergometrine 500 µg IV
c) Glycerine trinitrate 100 µg IV
d) Nifedipine 20 mg IV
e) Terbutaline 1 g IV

66

You see a 45-year-old nullipara in your gynaecology clinic who is a carrier for the BRCA1 mutation. She wishes to discuss surgery to reduce her cancer risk.

What is the approximate average cumulative risk of her developing ovarian-type cancer by the age of 70?

a) 10%
b) 25%
c) 40%
d) 55%
e) 70%

67

You examine a 28-year-old primigravid woman in the antenatal ward at 36 weeks of gestation with polymorphic eruption of pregnancy, associated with generalized urticarial papules and increasingly severe pruritus. It has not responded to emollient creams, systemic antihistamines or topical steroids.

What further treatment is most likely to be effective?

a) Emollient creams
b) Intravenous immunoglobulins
c) Systemic aciclovir
d) Systemic prednisolone
e) Ultraviolet B phototherapy

68

A primigravid woman is admitted for the medical management of early fetal demise at 15 weeks of gestation. She has received mifepristone 200 mg 48 hours prior to admission.

When prescribing her vaginal misoprostol, the total daily dosage should not exceed:

a) 400 µg
b) 800 µg
c) 1200 µg
d) 1600 µg
e) 2400 µg

69

A 40-year-old nulliparous woman is admitted with her fourth consecutive early pregnancy loss at 10 weeks of gestation.

A luteal-phase fall in which of these is associated with recurrent miscarriage?

a) Human chorionic gonadotrophin (hCG)
b) Insulin-like growth factor binding protein 1 (IGFBP1)
c) Oestradiol (E_2)
d) Prolactin (PRL)
e) Vitamin D

70

A 32-year-old nulliparous woman presents to the gynaecology ward with an incomplete miscarriage. This is now her third consecutive early pregnancy loss.

Which investigation should routinely be carried out?

a) Cervical length estimation
b) Chlamydia test
c) Cytogenetic analysis of the products of conception
d) Parental chromosome tests
e) Thyroid function tests

71

A 35-year-old woman attends your clinic for counselling regarding her risk of ovarian cancer. She has no family history of ovarian or breast cancer.

What is the lifetime risk of developing ovarian cancer in the general population?

a) < 1%
b) 1–2%
c) 3–4%
d) 5–6%
e) 7–8%

72

A 65-year-old woman is referred with an eight-month history of pain and itching in the vulval area. She is otherwise fit and well. You carry out a detailed clinical examination.

What appropriate investigation will you arrange to complement your clinical findings?

a) Blood tests and skin biopsy for all cases
b) Blood tests for autoimmune conditions if lichen planus is provisionally diagnosed
c) Blood tests for serum ferritin if vulval dermatitis is provisionally diagnosed
d) Blood tests for thyroid disorder and diabetes for all cases
e) Cervical smear if vulval intraepithelial neoplasia (VIN) is your clinical diagnosis

73

During the labour ward handover, the coordinator informs you that there is a 35-year-old para 1 woman in labour with a face presentation. A junior doctor, who wants to do postgraduate training in obstetrics and gynaecology, is keen to learn more about this presentation.

What is the engaging diameter in a face presentation?

a) Bitemporal diameter
b) Occipito-frontal diameter

c) Submento-bregmatic diameter
d) Suboccipito-bregmatic diameter
e) Vertico-mental diameter

74

A 26-year-old woman underwent surgical management of miscarriage and histopathology confirms normal trophoblast. Her last pregnancy, two years ago, was a molar pregnancy and she was followed up at the regional trophoblast screening centre.

What is the most appropriate follow-up, if any, in this pregnancy?

a) hCG level measurements in 4 weeks
b) hCG level measurements in 6 weeks
c) hCG level measurements monthly for 3 months
d) hCG level measurements monthly for 6 months
e) No follow-up

75

A 30-year-old primigravida presents in spontaneous labour at 41 weeks of gestation. On vaginal examination, the cervix is 8 cm dilated and the position of the vertex is left occipito-posterior.

What is the presenting diameter?

a) Bitemporal
b) Occipito-frontal
c) Submento-bregmatic
d) Suboccipito-bregmatic
e) Vertico-mental

76

You are attending a teaching session on labour management. You have been asked a series of questions regarding the mechanism by which the head is spontaneously born in a face presentation.

By what mechanism is the head delivered in a face presentation?

a) Extension
b) External rotation
c) Flexion
d) Internal rotation
e) Restitution

77

A 25-year-old woman requests emergency contraception following unprotected sexual intercourse on one occasion four days ago. She is currently taking a proton pump inhibitor for gastro-oesophageal reflux.

What emergency contraception would you recommend?

a) Copper intrauterine contraceptive device (IUCD)
b) Levonorgestrel (LNG)
c) LNG intrauterine system (Mirena coil)
d) Mifepristone
e) Ulipristal acetate (UPA)

78

A 25-year-old woman is referred by the sexual health clinic due to an adnexal mass detected during copper coil insertion. She is symptom-free. A transvaginal scan shows a simple left ovarian cyst of 63 × 65 mm.

What would be your management plan?

a) MRI
b) Perform CA-125
c) Perform CA-125, LDH, AFP, hCG
d) Ultrasound after 6 months
e) Ultrasound after 12 months

79

You are asked to see a 40-year-old woman referred by the urologist because of an incidental finding of a simple right ovarian cyst measuring 43 × 47 mm on pelvic ultrasound. She has no gynaecological complaints.

What is your management plan?

a) CA-125 assay
b) CT scan
c) Gynaecological review in 3 months
d) No follow-up
e) Repeat ultrasound scan in 6 months

80

A 23-year-old woman in her first pregnancy with a history of systemic lupus erythematosus (SLE) attends for a detailed fetal anomaly ultrasound at 20 weeks of gestation. Autoantibody profile has detected Sjögren's syndrome A/B (anti-Ro/anti-La) antibodies.

What is the risk of the fetus developing congenital heart block?

a) 2–3%
b) 5–6%
c) 8–9%
d) 11–12%
e) 14–15%

81

A pregnant patient with thalassaemia books at the high-risk antenatal clinic at 10 weeks of gestation. She has a history of splenectomy. Her platelet count at booking is 650×10^9/L.

When considering her thrombotic risk, what treatment would you currently advise during pregnancy?

a) Low-dose aspirin 75 mg/day
b) Low-dose aspirin 75 mg/day and low-molecular-weight heparin (LMWH) therapeutic dose
c) Low-dose aspirin 75 mg/day and LMWH thromboprophylaxis
d) Use of TED anti-embolism compression stockings
e) Use of TED anti-embolism compression stockings and low-dose aspirin 75 mg/day

82

A 35-year-old woman presents to the gynaecology clinic with left iliac fossa pain. Transvaginal ultrasound scan shows a 9 cm unilateral left ovarian mass, which is septated with echogenic foci. The right ovary cannot be identified separately and the uterus appears normal.

What are the most appropriate tumour markers to test in this case?

a) CA-125, AFP, hCG
b) CA-125, AFP, hCG, CEA
c) CA-125, AFP, hCG, LDH
d) CA-125, CEA, CA19-9
e) CA-125, CEA, LDH

83

The United Kingdom Medical Eligibility Criteria (UKMEC) offers guidance to clinicians when considering the use of contraceptives. There are four categories, with Category 1 being generally suitable and Category 4 completely contraindicated.

When considering the combined oral contraceptive pill, which of the following factors would be considered as a Category 4 contraindication (i.e. completely contraindicated)?

a) Age 30 and smoking (more than 35/day)
b) Family history of breast cancer with a known *BRCA* gene mutation
c) History of deep venous thrombosis (DVT)
d) Hypertension 140/90 mmHg
e) Three weeks postnatal and breastfeeding

84

A 28-year-old para 1 woman with a history of polycystic ovary syndrome presents to the gynaecology emergency unit with a six-hour history of severe, intermittent left iliac fossa pain, nausea, vomiting and low-grade pyrexia. Transvaginal ultrasound scan suggests an enlarged oedematous left ovary with abnormal colour Doppler flow. Her white cell count is 16×10^9/L (normal 4–11), C-reactive protein 70 mg/L (normal < 10). She has been fluid resuscitated and has received intramuscular opioid analgesia.

What is the ideal management for this woman?

a) Admit to the inpatient ward for close observation
b) Diagnostic laparoscopy and de-torsion of left ovary
c) Diagnostic laparoscopy and left oopherectomy
d) Diagnostic laparoscopy and left partial oopherectomy
e) Explorative laparotomy

85

A woman is readmitted 48 hours after a normal vaginal delivery. Symptoms and signs suggest profound septic shock.

What is the most appropriate first-line antibiotic regime to use?

a) Cefuroxime + metronidazole
b) Cefuroxime + metronidazole + gentamicin
c) Clindamycin + piperacillin/tazobactam
d) Co-amoxiclav + metronidazole
e) Co-amoxiclav + metronidazole + gentamicin

86

A 29-year-old woman is brought in to the emergency department by paramedics with a suspected pelvic fracture at 34 weeks of gestation after being hit by a car. She is hypotensive and tachycardic. She is being fluid resuscitated, and bloods including crossmatch have been sent.

What is the priority in the management of this woman?

a) Commence fetal monitoring in resuscitation
b) Immobilize the pelvis
c) Perform a full primary survey
d) Plan pelvic imaging and orthopaedic review
e) Plan transfer to labour ward for immediate delivery of baby

87

A 47-year-old woman had a total abdominal hysterectomy for fibroids. Intraoperatively, deep retractor blades were used. She presents seven days postoperatively with weakness of hip flexion and adduction and knee extension. There is unilateral loss of knee jerk reflex and loss of sensation over the anteromedial thigh.

Which nerve is likely to have been injured intraoperatively?

a) Femoral nerve
b) Genitofemoral nerve
c) Ilioinguinal nerve
d) Lateral cutaneous nerve of the thigh
e) Obturator nerve

88

A 38-week pregnant para 0 + 0 calls the maternity assessment department for advice. Her husband has been diagnosed with herpes zoster and she thinks she has not had chickenpox in the past.

What is the most appropriate management for this woman?

a) Check serology for varicella immunity
b) Give varicella-zoster immunoglobulin (VZIG)
c) Prescribe a course of aciclovir treatment
d) Reassure patient that she does not require treatment
e) Varicella vaccination

89

A 34-year-old woman is admitted for a diagnostic laparoscopy to investigate subfertility. She weighs 65 kg and is fit and healthy. The trainee performing the procedure is under direct supervision by the consultant.

At what angle to the skin should the primary trocar be inserted?

a) 15°
b) 30°
c) 45°
d) 60°
e) 90°

90

A 28-year-old woman undergoes surgical termination of pregnancy at 13 weeks of gestation and sustains a uterine perforation.

Which one of the following is the instrument most commonly causing perforation?

a) Curette
b) Hegar dilator
c) Sponge-holding forceps
d) Suction cannula
e) Uterine sound

91

An 85-year-old woman has recently been diagnosed with vaginal carcinoma. The histology report confirmed squamous cell vaginal carcinoma and high prevalence of human papillomavirus (HPV).

Which type of HPV is responsible for the majority of vaginal carcinomas?

a) HPV-16
b) HPV-18
c) HPV-31
d) HPV-33
e) HPV-35

92

A 28-year-old woman is in her third pregnancy. She is admitted for induction of labour for postdates. She is a known asthmatic and was admitted two weeks ago with exacerbation of asthma.

Which one of the following medications can be used safely for management of labour and postpartum?

a) Diclofenac
b) Ergometrine
c) Prostaglandin E_2
d) Prostaglandin $F_{2\alpha}$
e) Syntometrine

93

Highly active antiretroviral therapy (HAART) in now routine in the management of HIV-positive women in pregnancy and is very effective in reducing mother-to-child transmission (MTCT) of HIV.

What is the incidence of transmission reduced to?

a) 0.1–0.5%
b) 1–2%
c) 3–5%
d) 6–8%
e) 9–11%

94

A 34-year-old nulliparous woman with asthma attends the antenatal clinic at 11 weeks of gestation. She is currently on regular salbutamol and steroid inhalers. She enquires regarding the effect of pregnancy on her asthma.

At what stage of pregnancy are exacerbations of asthma most common?

a) < 24 weeks
b) 24–36 weeks
c) > 36 weeks
d) During labour
e) In the postpartum period

95

A 28-year-old woman had a caesarean section for failure to progress. She visits her general practitioner four months postpartum with paraesthesia and sharp burning pains radiating from the incision site to the left labia and thigh.

Which nerve is most likely to have been involved?

a) Femoral nerve
b) Genitofemoral nerve
c) Iliohypogastric nerve
d) Lateral cutaneous nerve
e) Obturator nerve

96

A 31-year-old nulliparous woman with HbSS is considering having a child with her partner, who has HbAS.

What is the probability that the child will have sickle cell disease?

a) 25%
b) 33%
c) 50%
d) 75%
e) 100%

97

A 29-year-old woman presents at 10 weeks of gestation with persistent vaginal bleeding and severe hyperemesis. On examination, the uterus is equivalent to 16 weeks in size. Ultrasound scan suggests a molar pregnancy. Uterine evacuation is performed under ultrasound guidance. She is registered to a UK screening centre to follow her gestational trophoblastic disease (GTD).

What is the optimum follow-up for GTD?

a) If human chorionic gonadotrophin (hCG) has reverted to normal within 28 days, follow-up will be for 6 months
b) If hCG has reverted to normal within 28 days, follow-up will be for 9 months
c) If hCG has reverted to normal within 28 days, follow-up will be for 12 months
d) If hCG has reverted to normal within 56 days, follow-up will be for 6 months
e) If hCG has reverted to normal within 56 days, follow-up will be for 9 months

98

A 41-year-old woman presents at 36 weeks of gestation in active labour. She has had a previous caesarean section and a subsequent precipitate vaginal delivery.

An ultrasound scan at 20 weeks showed a bilobed low-lying placenta. A repeat ultrasound scan at 32 weeks revealed a normally located placenta with polyhydramnios. Immediately after rupture of membranes, she started bleeding vaginally with associated cardiotocography (CTG) abnormalities.

What is the most likely diagnosis?

a) Abruptio placentae
b) Placenta accreta
c) Placenta percreta
d) Placenta praevia
e) Vasa praevia

99

A 28-year-old woman presents at 35 weeks in her second pregnancy feeling unwell, with backache, fever and rigors. She has a temperature of 39.5 °C. Her blood pressure is 60/40 mmHg, respiratory rate is 44 breaths/minute, pulse rate is 145 bpm. Speculum examination confirms foul-smelling vaginal discharge, and the serum lactate is > 4 mmol/L. She is not responding to the routine resuscitative measures.

What is the risk of maternal mortality?

a) 30%
b) 40%
c) 50%
d) 60%
e) 70%

100

A diagnostic laparoscopy is being performed on a patient for suspected perforation of the uterus during suction evacuation of retained products of conception.

What is the most common site of uterine perforation?

a) Anterior
b) Fundus
c) Left lateral
d) Posterior
e) Right lateral

101

A 38-year-old woman has undergone a difficult laparoscopically assisted vaginal hysterectomy, with blood loss of 600 mL. Forty-eight hours after surgery, she complains of flank pain and has abdominal distension with generalized abdominal tenderness. She has oliguria and she is apyrexial. Bowel sounds are present but scanty. Investigations have revealed haemoglobin 10.8 g/L (normal 11.5–16.5), white cell count 8.3×10^9/L (normal 4–11) and creatinine 342 µmol/L (normal 27–88).

What is the most likely diagnosis?

a) Bowel injury
b) Ureteric injury
c) Urinary tract infection
d) Vault haematoma
e) Wound infection

102

You are asked to review a woman eight hours after a vaginal delivery. She has an Obstetric Modified Early Warning Score of 6, which four hours previously was 0. She is tachycardic, tachypnoeic, hypotensive and pyrexial. She has abdominal tenderness and a sore throat.

What is the most likely causative organism?

a) *Clostridium septicum*
b) *Escherichia coli*
c) Group A *Streptococcus*
d) *Haemophilus influenzae*
e) *Staphylococcus aureus*

103

You are investigating the effect of promoting immediate skin-to-skin contact at elective caesarean section and breastfeeding rates at six weeks postpartum. You have collected data over a period of six months on whether babies had immediate skin-to-skin contact and whether they were still being breastfed at six weeks.

What is the single most likely statistical test you would apply to the data to find a difference between the two groups?

a) ANOVA
b) Chi-squared
c) Odds ratio
d) Pearson's correlation
e) Student's *t*-test

104

A 30-year-old nulliparous woman has a cervical smear taken at her general practitioner's surgery as part of her routine screening recall. The result of the smear shows mild dyskaryosis. This is her first abnormal smear.

What is the appropriate management?

a) Offer prophylactic vaccination
b) Refer to a colposcopy clinic
c) Refer to a colposcopy clinic if she tests positive for high-risk HPV
d) Repeat the smear in 6 months
e) Repeat the smear in 24 months

105

A 34-year-old primigravida presents at 28 weeks of gestation with fever and flu-like symptoms with no gastrointestinal symptoms. She gives a history of recent travel to sub-Saharan Africa. Investigations confirm < 2% red blood cells parasitized with *Plasmodium falciparum*. She is clinically stable with no signs of severe infection. She has no drug allergies.

What is the most appropriate drug regime used for initial treatment?

a) Intravenous artesunate 2.4 mg/kg at 0, 12 and 24 hours followed by daily doses
b) Intravenous quinine 10 mg/kg TDS + IV clindamycin 450 mg TDS
c) Intravenous quinine 20 mg/kg loading dose followed by 10 mg/kg TDS + IV clindamycin 450 mgTDS
d) Oral quinine 600 mg followed by 300 mg 6–8 hours later
e) Oral quinine 600 mg TDS + oral clindamycin 450 mg TDS

106

A 70-year-old woman had a sacrospinous fixation one week ago. She was readmitted complaining of severe right buttock and perineal pain, which is aggravated in the seating position.

What is the most likely nerve involvement?

a) Common peroneal nerve
b) Genitofemoral nerve
c) Ilioinguinal nerve
d) Obturator nerve
e) Pudendal nerve

107

A 24-year-old primigravida presents at 24 weeks with increasing shortness of breath, orthopnoea and paroxysmal nocturnal dyspnoea. This was an unplanned pregnancy. She is known to have thalassaemia major, and her last blood transfusion was one week ago. Her current haemoglobin is 100 g/L.

Which is the most appropriate investigation for her?

a) Arterial blood gas (ABG)
b) Cardiac magnetic resonance imaging (MRI)
c) CT-guided pulmonary angiogram (CTPA)
d) Echocardiogram (ECHO)
e) Ventilation/perfusion scan (V/Q scan)

108

A 39-year-old woman has been referred with a history of three consecutive miscarriages. The first two miscarriages occurred before 10 weeks and the third was at 13 weeks of gestation. She has no significant medical history, and no uterine abnormalities were identified on a pelvic ultrasound scan.

What is the risk of miscarriage in the next pregnancy for this woman?

a) < 10%
b) 15–25%
c) 30–40%
d) 45–50%
e) 55–60%

109

A 29-year-old nulliparous woman, suffering from cystic fibrosis, is contemplating pregnancy. Her sister-in-law recently had a baby with cystic fibrosis. Her partner is detected to be a carrier for cystic fibrosis.

What is the risk of the baby having cystic fibrosis?

a) 1/2
b) 1/4
c) 1/8
d) 1/25
e) 1/40

110

A 41-year-old primigravida is 14 weeks pregnant. She had in-vitro fertilization (IVF) and has a dichorionic and diamniotic twin pregnancy. She has chronic kidney disease and is attending the antenatal clinic for her first medical appointment.

Which one of her risk factors is the strongest predisposition for pre-eclampsia?

a) Age > 40 years
b) Chronic kidney disease
c) First pregnancy
d) IVF pregnancy
e) Multiple pregnancy

111

A 53-year-old woman had a total abdominal hysterectomy with bilateral salpingo-oophorectomy and omentectomy for a suspicious large ovarian cyst with raised CA-125. At laparotomy, it was noted that the tumour was limited to one ovary, but the capsule was breached. It was staged as Ic ovarian adenocarcinoma. The cytology for peritoneal washings was positive for adenocarcinoma cells.

What is the five-year survival?

a) 20%
b) 40%
c) 60%
d) 80%
e) 90%

112

A 27-year-old woman attends antenatal clinic at 29 weeks of gestation and is found to have a blood pressure of 148/99 mmHg. Testing her urine shows ++ of proteinuria. She is asymptomatic.

What is the most appropriate initial management?

a) Admit to hospital for observation
b) Arrange for the community midwife to visit the patient at home in 24 hours
c) Commence methyldopa 250 mg three times a day and follow up on day assessment unit in 48 hours
d) Commence treatment with labetalol 200 mg three times a day and follow up on day assessment unit in 48 hours
e) Refer to day assessment unit for blood pressure profile and further assessment

113

A 30-year-old woman had a 3c perineal tear at her first vaginal delivery. She attends the postnatal perineal trauma clinic at six weeks. She is concerned about her persistent symptom of faecal urgency.

What percentage of women are asymptomatic at 12 months after sustaining a third-degree tear?

a) 1–20%
b) 21–40%
c) 41–60%
d) 61–80%
e) 81–100%

114

A 49-year-old woman attends the urogynaecology clinic with symptoms of frequency, urgency and nocturia. She has already had bladder training. Her urinalysis is negative for infection.

What of the following is the next level of management?

a) Mirabegron
b) Pelvic floor exercises
c) Sacral nerve stimulation
d) Trospium
e) Urodynamic investigations

115

A low-risk primigravida is admitted in spontaneous labour at term with intact membranes. She is contracting strongly, four in 10 minutes. The cervix is effaced and 5 cm dilated, cephalic presentation, occipito-anterior position with no caput or moulding and 1 cm above the ischial spines. Four hours later, she is 6 cm dilated. All other findings are unchanged. Intermittent auscultation is normal.

According to National Institute for Health and Care Excellence (NICE) guidance, what is the diagnosis and recommended management?

a) Adequate progress in the first stage, vaginal examination in 4 hours
b) Confirmed delay in the first stage, amniotomy and vaginal examination in 2 hours
c) Confirmed delay in the first stage, amniotomy and vaginal examination in 4 hours
d) Suspected delay in the first stage, amniotomy and vaginal examination in 2 hours
e) Suspected delay in the first stage, amniotomy and vaginal examination in 4 hours

116

A 90-year-old woman with multiple comorbidities has a vault prolapse that cannot be managed with a shelf pessary. She is struggling with the repeated hospital visits and examinations and requests definitive treatment.

Which surgical procedure is best suited to this woman?

a) Abdominal sacrocolpopexy
b) Burch colposuspension
c) Colpocleisis
d) Posterior intravaginal slingplasty
e) Vaginal uterosacral ligament suspension

117

A 45-year-old woman is due to have a transobturator tape procedure for stress urinary incontinence. You counsel her about the risks of the procedure, including the risk of obturator nerve injury.

What motor findings would be consistent with obturator nerve injury?

a) Weakness of hip extension
b) Weakness of hip external rotation
c) Weakness of hip flexion
d) Weakness of thigh abduction
e) Weakness of thigh adduction

118

A 30-year-old primiparous woman attends pre-conception counselling prior to undergoing in-vitro fertilization (IVF) treatment, because of a strong family history of venous thromboembolism in several first-degree relatives. She has a body mass index (BMI) of 34 and has no previous major medical problems.

Which blood test would be most helpful in determining her management?

a) Anti-Xa levels
b) Anticardiolipin antibodies
c) Lupus anticoagulant
d) Methyltetrahydrofolate reductase genotype
e) Thrombophilia screen

119

A 29-year-old primigravida presents with an intrauterine fetal death at 26 weeks. She has been feeling unwell for a few days. She has intact membranes but the liquor is noted to be green at delivery.

What is the most likely cause of this fetal loss?

a) Cytomegalovirus
b) Group A *Streptococcus*
c) Group B *Streptococcus*
d) *Listeria monocytogenes*
e) Parvovirus B19

120

A 35-year-old woman with known myasthenia gravis attends for pre-conception counselling.

Which of the following drugs should be avoided in pregnancy?

a) Azathioprine
b) Ciclosporin
c) Mycophenolate mofetil
d) Prednisolone
e) Pyridostigmine

121

A 27-year-old woman presents in labour having had no antenatal care in the UK. She informs the midwife that she is HIV positive. She has had no antiretroviral treatment in her pregnancy.

What is the risk of vertical transmission with no intervention in this case?

a) 5–10%
b) 15–20%

c) 25–30%
d) 35–40%
e) 45–50%

122

A 49-year-old woman attends for outpatient hysteroscopy to investigate abnormal vaginal bleeding.

What intervention is routinely recommended to reduce procedure-related pain?

a) Dihydrocodeine pre-procedure
b) Instillation of local anaesthetic gel into the cervical canal pre-procedure
c) Misoprostol pre-procedure
d) Non-steroidal anti-inflammatory drugs pre-procedure
e) Paracervical block with local anaesthetic pre-procedure

123

A 58-year-old postmenopausal woman presents with pelvic pain and a persistent 6 cm simple unilocular left ovarian cyst on pelvic ultrasound. Her CA-125 is 25 IU/mL. She opts for surgical management.

What is the most appropriate surgical management?

a) Aspiration of the cyst
b) Bilateral oophorectomy
c) Left oophorectomy
d) Left ovarian cystectomy
e) Total hysterectomy, bilateral salpingo-oophorectomy and omentectomy

124

A 46-year-old woman had a total abdominal hysterectomy for heavy menstrual bleeding due to fibroids. She had defaulted many years ago from the routine recall for cervical smears but this was not picked up before the operation. Histology showed no cervical intraepithelial neoplasia (CIN) in the hysterectomy specimen.

What is the most appropriate follow-up?

a) No further cytology required
b) Vaginal vault cytology immediately
c) Vaginal vault cytology at 6 weeks
d) Vaginal vault cytology at 6 months
e) Vaginal vault cytology at 6 months and 18 months

125

A 20-year-old primigravida has an incidental finding of cervical length of 20 mm at her routine 20-week anomaly scan. She is asymptomatic and has no significant past medical or surgical history.

What is the most appropriate management?

a) Abdominal cerclage
b) Cervical cerclage
c) Counsel the woman that no further action is required
d) Progesterone pessaries
e) Serial ultrasound scan to assess cervical length

126

A primigravid woman has been having serial ultrasound scans for a small-for-gestational-age fetus. The fetal biometry is below the 10th centile, with normal liquor volumes and umbilical artery Doppler. She reports good fetal movements. She is currently 37 weeks pregnant and has declined induction of labour.

After appropriate counselling regarding risks to her baby, what is the most appropriate management for this woman?

a) Admit her for observation
b) Cardiotocography weekly
c) Cardiotocography twice weekly
d) Umbilical artery Doppler and liquor volume weekly
e) Umbilical artery Doppler and liquor volume twice weekly

127

A 36-year-old woman has attended for pre-conception counselling. She has a history of systemic lupus erythematosus for the last 15 years. Her first child, now two years old, had a pacemaker fitted for congenital heart block.

What is the risk of heart block in subsequent pregnancy?

a) 5%
b) 15%
c) 25%
d) 35%
e) 50%

128

A 25-year-old woman attends the postnatal clinic. She delivered her son eight weeks ago at 27 weeks of gestation following an eclamptic seizure. She is keen to have further children.

What is her risk of pre-eclampsia in her next pregnancy?

a) 5%
b) 10%
c) 25%
d) 50%
e) 75%

129

A 25-year-old pregnant woman with sickle cell disease and a history of previous transfusion is blood group B negative. She has anti-D antibodies. She requires a non-emergency blood transfusion.

Which blood would be suitable for transfusion?

a) B negative, CMV negative, Kell negative
b) B negative, CMV negative, Kell positive
c) B negative, CMV positive, Kell positive
d) B positive, CMV negative, Kell negative
e) B positive, CMV positive, Kell positive

130

A 35-year-old woman is admitted to hospital at 34 weeks of gestation with a worsening of her asthma.

Approximately what proportion of women experience a deterioration of their asthma in pregnancy?

a) 10%
b) 30%
c) 50%
d) 60%
e) 75%

131

A 27-year-old woman with epilepsy attends antenatal clinic in the third trimester of pregnancy. She is well controlled on lamotrigine.

In women with treated epilepsy, what is the risk of having a tonic–clonic seizure in the peripartum period?

a) 1–5%
b) 10–15%
c) 20–25%
d) 30–35%
e) 40–45%

132

A 24-year-old woman in her first pregnancy has been diagnosed with hydrops fetalis on her anomaly scan at 20 weeks of gestation. Maternal serology is negative for immune causes.

What is the risk of fetal mortality without intervention in non-immune hydrops fetalis?

a) 20%
b) 40%
c) 60%
d) 80%
e) 100%

133

You are working as a year 4 specialist trainee. You have a meeting with your educational supervisor in which your achievements and challenges over the last four months are discussed. You jointly plan specific objectives to achieve over the next four months, including a clinical audit and attending a postgraduate course.

How would you best describe this encounter?

a) Appraisal
b) Mini clinical evaluation exercise
c) Revalidation
d) Summative assessment
e) Team observation

134

A 22-year-old woman is on the postnatal ward having had a normal delivery. The midwife notices that the baby has sticky eyes on the morning after delivery.

What is the most common causative organism of infective neonatal conjunctivitis?

a) *Chlamydia trachomatis*
b) *Haemophilus influenzae*
c) *Neisseria gonorrhoeae*
d) *Staphylococcus aureus*
e) *Streptococcus pneumoniae*

135

Following instrumental vaginal delivery, vaginal and rectal examination shows a perineal tear involving less than 50% of the external anal sphincter. The internal anal sphincter and rectal mucosa are intact.

What is the classification of this perineal injury?

a) Second degree
b) Third degree: 3a
c) Third degree: 3b
d) Third degree: 3c
e) Fourth degree

136

You have performed a diagnostic hysteroscopy which was complicated by a uterine perforation. You complete a clinical adverse incident report and later review the case to identify any gaps in your knowledge or skills. You record and discuss your thoughts with your educational supervisor.

How would you best describe this learning exercise?

a) Appraisal
b) Mini clinical evaluation exercise
c) Reflective practice
d) Risk assessment
e) Root cause analysis

137

You are performing a diagnostic laparoscopy. You have placed the primary trocar following carbon dioxide insufflation with a Veress needle.

What is the recommended range of intra-abdominal pressure for insertion of the secondary trocar under direct vision?

a) 5–10 mmHg
b) 10–15 mmHg
c) 15–20 mmHg
d) 20–25 mmHg
e) 25–30 mmHg

138

A 23-year-old woman undergoes a surgical evacuation for a suspected molar pregnancy. Histology has confirmed a partial mole.

What is the most common chromosomal composition of a partial mole?

a) 1 paternal and 1 maternal gametes
b) 1 paternal and 2 maternal gametes
c) 2 paternal and 1 maternal gametes
d) 2 paternal and no maternal gametes
e) 3 paternal and 1 maternal gametes

139

A 60-year-old postmenopausal woman presents to the gynaecology clinic with a history of gradual onset of vulval itching and burning. She has suffered from urinary incontinence for two years. Examination reveals vulval erythema and scaling.

What is the most likely diagnosis?

a) Irritant dermatitis
b) Lichen planus
c) Lichen sclerosus
d) Paget's disease
e) Squamous cell carcinoma

140

A 31-year-old woman is diagnosed with a missed miscarriage at 11 weeks in her first pregnancy. Her body mass index (BMI) is 26 and she has no medical history. She wants to know the reason for the miscarriage.

What is the most common cause of first-trimester miscarriage?

a) Fetal aneuploidy
b) Infection
c) Smoking
d) Thrombophilia
e) Uterine anomaly

141

A 39-year-old woman has a normal delivery of her third baby. She requests long-term contraception. She has previously used a copper intrauterine device but has a history of menorrhagia. You counsel her about a levonorgestrel-releasing intrauterine system (Mirena coil).

What is the recommended time interval for insertion of the levonorgestrel-releasing system following delivery?

a) 7 days
b) 14 days
c) 21 days
d) 28 days
e) 42 days

142

A 26-year-old woman has pelvic girdle pain and has been booked for induction of labour at 39 weeks. She is diagnosed with primary varicella-zoster virus at 38 + 6 weeks of gestation.

What would you recommend to reduce the risk of neonatal varicella infection?

a) Delay her induction for a week
b) Deliver by elective caesarean section
c) Intravenous aciclovir for the neonate
d) Intravenous aciclovir in labour
e) Oral aciclovir for the mother from diagnosis

143

A 32-year-old primigravida is admitted in spontaneous labour with confirmed ruptured membranes at 39 weeks of gestation. Her temperature is 38.5 °C.

In this case, what is the estimated risk of early-onset neonatal group B streptococcal (EOGBS) disease?

a) 1/10
b) 1/20
c) 1/100
d) 1/200
e) 1/1000

144

A 29-year-old woman is referred to the gynaecology clinic with a history of recurrent first-trimester miscarriages. Initial investigations were negative for anticardiolipin antibodies and lupus anticoagulant. She has no other medical problems. Previous cytogenetic analysis on products of conception showed normal fetal karyotype.

Which one of the following investigations should be recommended next?

a) Hysteroscopy
b) Inherited thrombophilia screen
c) LH/FSH ratio
d) Parental karyotyping
e) Ultrasound scan of pelvis

145

A 29-year-old woman presents with a history of heavy vaginal bleeding two weeks after having a normal vaginal birth. Clinical assessment indicates retained products of conception, and she is consented for surgical evacuation of retained products of conception (ERPC).

What is the risk of uterine perforation in this case?

a) 1%
b) 5%
c) 10%
d) 15%
e) 20%

146

A woman is being treated with magnesium sulphate for severe pre-eclampsia. There is concern about magnesium toxicity.

What is the first sign of magnesium toxicity?

a) Bradycardia
b) Decreased urine output
c) Loss of deep tendon reflexes
d) Reduced consciousness
e) Respiratory depression

147

A couple presented with a history of primary infertility. The male partner has cystic fibrosis, and semen analysis showed azoospermia.

What is the most likely cause of azoospermia in this patient?

a) Congenital absence of ejaculatory duct
b) Congenital bilateral absence of seminal vesicles
c) Congenital bilateral absence of vas deferens
d) Obstruction following genitourinary infection
e) Retrograde ejaculation

148

A 20-year-old woman has had side effects to various hormonal contraceptives. She is not keen on intrauterine devices. She wants to try a cervical cap with spermicide.

What is the optimum duration of application for a cervical cap for it to be most effective?

a) Insert just before intercourse and remove immediately
b) Insert just before intercourse and remove after 6 hours
c) Insert an hour before intercourse and remove an hour after
d) Insert an hour before intercourse and remove after 3 hours
e) Insert an hour before intercourse and remove after 12 hours

149

A 25-year-old woman intending to commence the combined contraceptive pill wishes to discuss the risk of venous thromboembolism (VTE). She has no other risk factors for VTE.

Which progestogen in combined oral contraceptives is associated with the lowest risk of VTE?

a) Desogestrel
b) Drospirenone
c) Etonogestrel
d) Gestodene
e) Norgestimate

150

A 25-year-old primiparous woman had a second-trimester miscarriage at 16 weeks. She had painless dilatation of cervix followed by rupture of membranes. There is no history of cervical surgery.

What is the most appropriate management for future pregnancy?

a) Abdominal cerclage pre-pregnancy
b) Cervical cerclage at 13–15 weeks

c) Clinical assessment of cervical length at 14 weeks
d) Pre-pregnancy assessment of cervical length
e) Serial sonographic surveillance of cervical length in pregnancy

151

A 39-year-old primigravida is 33 weeks pregnant. She reports to the day assessment unit with a second episode of reduced fetal movements. Initial examination and cardiotocography (CTG) are normal.

What is the most appropriate next step?

a) Deliver baby following a course of steroids
b) Reassure her and provide her with a kick chart
c) Repeat CTG in 2 days
d) Ultrasound scan
e) Umbilical artery Doppler study

152

A 28-year-old in her first pregnancy has delivered normally and has had early cord clamping and 10 IU of oxytocin IM and controlled cord traction applied. The placenta has not delivered yet.

After how long would you call it a prolonged third stage of labour?

a) 10 minutes
b) 20 minutes
c) 30 minutes
d) 45 minutes
e) 60 minutes

153

A 16-year-old girl presents with primary amenorrhoea. She is examined and found to have normal secondary sexual characteristics but a small blind-ending vagina. Ultrasound scan reveals normal ovaries, and she has normal XX chromosomes on karyotyping.

What condition does this girl most likely have?

a) 5-Alpha-reductase type 2 deficiency
b) Complete androgen insensitivity syndrome
c) Congenital adrenal hyperplasia (CAH)
d) Mayer–Rokitansky–Küster–Hauser (MRKH) syndrome
e) Swyer's syndrome

154

A 24-year-old woman presents to the emergency department with light vaginal bleeding after five weeks of amenorrhoea. A recent pregnancy test was positive. She also complains of sharp pain in the left iliac fossa. Blood tests reveal that she is O negative blood group.

Which subsequent outcome would require anti-D prophylaxis?

a) Complete miscarriage
b) Expectant management of early fetal demise

c) Medical management of ectopic pregnancy
d) Medical management of miscarriage
e) Surgical management of ectopic pregnancy

155

You are taking consent from a primigravida for an elective caesarean section for major placenta praevia. You explain that one of the serious risks associated with the procedure is massive obstetric haemorrhage.

Which of the following best represents the risk of massive obstetric haemorrhage in this woman?

a) 5 in 100
b) 10 in 100
c) 20 in 100
d) 30 in 100
e) 50 in 100

156

A 28-year-old primigravida at 38 weeks of gestation presents with a history of rupture of membranes six hours ago. She is apyrexial, is not having any contractions, and is confirmed to be draining clear liquor. While writing your notes, you discover that she has been recently treated for a group B streptococcal urinary tract infection.

What should you offer her next?

a) Augmentation of labour and prophylactic intravenous antibiotics in 24 hours
b) Augmentation of labour and prophylactic intravenous antibiotics immediately
c) Augmentation of labour immediately and intravenous antibiotics when contracting
d) Intravenous antibiotics with the onset of active labour
e) Prophylactic intravenous antibiotics immediately and await events

157

You are teaching a midwife how to perform McRoberts' manoeuvre.

Which of the following best describes McRoberts' manoeuvre?

a) Extension and abduction of maternal hips
b) Extension and adduction of maternal hips
c) Flexion and abduction of maternal hips
d) Flexion and abduction of maternal knees
e) Flexion and adduction of maternal hips

158

A 25-year-old man was referred with a history of secondary subfertility. Semen analysis confirmed azoospermia on two separate occasions two months apart. His initial hormone profile indicated reduced follicle-stimulating hormone (FSH) (0.6 IU/L) and luteinizing hormone (LH) (0.8 IU/L) concentrations.

What condition is the most likely explanation?

a) Cystic fibrosis carrier
b) Klinefelter syndrome
c) Taking anabolic steroids
d) Taking azathioprine
e) Varicocele

159

A 25-year-old woman attends your clinic for review. She presents with three unexplained first-trimester miscarriages.

What is the estimated miscarriage rate in her next pregnancy?

a) 20%
b) 30%
c) 40%
d) 50%
e) 60%

160

You are teaching a group of medical students on maternal obesity. They would like to know the impact of obesity on pregnant women.

As reported by the Centre for Maternal and Child Enquiries (CMACE) for the years 2006–08, what percentage of maternal deaths involved women who were obese?

a) 5–10%
b) 11–15%
c) 16–20%
d) 21–25%
e) 26–30%

161

A 22-year-old woman attends her postnatal review six weeks after the delivery of her first child. She has had an emergency caesarean section at 33 weeks of gestation for severe pre-eclampsia complicated with HELLP syndrome.

What is her risk of developing pre-eclampsia in her next pregnancy?

a) 1 in 2
b) 1 in 4
c) 1 in 6
d) 1 in 8
e) 1 in 10

162

A woman known to be a group B *Streptococcus* (GBS) carrier in her current pregnancy presents with a history of rupture of membranes at 33 weeks of gestation. She is well and is not in established labour. Her previous child was admitted to the neonatal unit and treated with antibiotics for confirmed neonatal GBS infection at birth.

What is the most appropriate next step in her management, once you have confirmed rupture of membranes?

a) Administer steroids and observe
b) Administer steroids, commence intravenous benzylpenicillin and induce labour in 24 hours
c) Administer steroids, commence intravenous benzylpenicillin and observe
d) Administer steroids, commence oral erythromycin and induce labour in 24 hours
e) Administer steroids, commence oral erythromycin and observe

163

You are counselling a primigravida with a breech presentation at 37 weeks of gestation for external cephalic version (ECV).

What is the rate of spontaneous version in this woman if ECV is not performed?

a) 2%
b) 5%
c) 8%
d) 11%
e) 14%

164

A 38-year-old woman attends your antenatal clinic. She is known to carry monochorionic twins. At 28 weeks, one of the twins unfortunately dies in utero. The woman wants to know the risk of death of the surviving twin in the event of the pregnancy continuing.

What is the risk of death of the co-twin?

a) 12%
b) 22%
c) 32%
d) 42%
e) 52%

165

The midwife in the clinic shows you a blood result of a woman booked under you. The result shows she has anti-D antibodies. She is 24 weeks into her second pregnancy. The first was a term birth and the baby was well.

What titre of anti-D level would prompt you to refer the patient to a fetal medicine specialist?

a) Anti-D levels: 0.5 IU/mL
b) Anti-D levels: 1.5 IU/mL
c) Anti-D levels: 2.5 IU/mL
d) Anti-D levels: 3.5 IU/mL
e) Anti-D levels: 4.5 IU/mL

166

A 60-year-old woman presents to your gynaecology clinic with a history of recurrent urinary tract infection (UTI) and symptoms of utero-vaginal prolapse.

Which of the following is a description of recurrent UTI?

a) At least two UTIs over a 12-month period
b) At least three UTIs over a 12-month period
c) At least four UTIs over a 12-month period
d) At least five UTIs over a 12-month period
e) At least six UTIs over a 12-month period

167

A 15-year-old girl presents with primary amenorrhoea although her secondary sexual characteristics are normally developed. She complains of having cyclical lower abdominal pain over the previous six months.

What is the most likely diagnosis?

a) Androgen insensitivity syndrome
b) Constitutional delay
c) Hyperprolactinaemia
d) Imperforate hymen
e) Pregnancy

168

A 28-year-old nulliparous woman presents to your gynaecology clinic with a history of infrequent periods occurring every three to four months since menarche at 13. Her body mass index (BMI) is 32. She suffers from mild asthma and has no other medical or surgical history of note.

What is the most likely cause for her presentation?

a) Excessive physical exercise
b) Hyperthyroidism
c) Ovarian cysts
d) Polycystic ovary syndrome
e) Prolactinoma

169

A woman had a difficult abdominal hysterectomy for a fibroid uterus. The transverse suprapubic incision needed to be extended laterally on both sides to facilitate the surgery. Postoperatively she developed sharp, burning pain and paraesthesia over her mons pubis, labia and the lateral aspect of her thigh. On examination, no motor weakness is found.

Which nerve is affected?

a) Femoral
b) Genitofemoral
c) Ilioinguinal
d) Lateral cutaneous nerve of the thigh
e) Obturator

170

An 89-year-old woman is reviewed in the urogynaecology clinic. She complains of increased frequency of urination, urgency, urge incontinence and nocturia. Her symptoms are disturbing her quality of life. She is very frail and does not wish to have any surgical intervention.

Which of the following is the most appropriate first-line treatment for the management of her symptoms?

a) Duloxetine
b) Mirabegron
c) Oxybutynin
d) Solifenacin
e) Tolterodine

171

A 39-year-old woman is booked at 10 weeks of gestation in her second pregnancy. She was referred to a consultant-led antenatal clinic, because her booking blood test detected anti-c antibodies at a titre of 5.4 IU/mL.

What is the most appropriate antenatal management plan for this woman with regard to anti-c antibodies?

a) Anti-c levels should be measured every 4 weeks until delivery
b) Anti-c levels should be measured every 4 weeks up to 28 weeks of gestation and then every 2 weeks until delivery
c) Anti-c levels should be measured every 6 weeks up to 34 weeks of gestation and then every 2 weeks until delivery
d) Monitoring of anti-c levels is indicated only when anti-c levels are > 7.5 IU/mL at booking
e) Referral to a fetal medicine specialist is indicated, as anti-c titres do not correlate well with either the development or the severity of fetal anaemia

172

A 27-year-old woman with a history of spinal cord injury (SCI) attends a pre-conception clinic along with her husband. This clinic is run by an obstetrician specializing in SCI in pregnancy. A care plan is discussed with this couple, based on the woman's disability and available support. The consultant informs them about autonomic dysreflexia, which is a potentially dangerous medical emergency in such cases.

Autonomic dysreflexia may develop in individuals with a neurological level of spinal cord injury:

a) Above the second lumbar vertebral level (L2)
b) At or above the fourth thoracic vertebral level (T4)
c) At or above the sixth thoracic vertebral level (T6)
d) At or above the twelfth thoracic vertebral level (T12)
e) Below the tenth thoracic vertebral level (T10)

173

The consultant is asked to review a woman at 22 weeks of gestation, as her ultrasound scan suggests that the fetus has an echogenic bowel. The results of cytomegalovirus (CMV) tests performed two weeks previously indicate that she seroconverted in the previous three months. The samples were tested in parallel at the regional laboratory.

What is the risk of vertical transmission of CMV?

a) 10%
b) 20%
c) 30%
d) 40%
e) 50%

174

A primigravida presents at 33 weeks of gestation with a history of itching involving the palms and soles of the feet for one week. On examination, she has evidence of dermatographia artefacta. Her liver functions show modest elevation of both aspartate transaminase (AST) and alanine transaminase (ALT), and a normal bilirubin. There is no evidence of a rash.

What is the most likely clinical diagnosis?

a) Atopic eruption of pregnancy
b) Chronic active hepatitis
c) Pemphigoid gestationis

d) Obstetric cholestasis
e) Polymorphic eruption of pregnancy

175

A woman at 28 weeks of gestation has been in contact with her neighbour who developed chickenpox two days ago. She is unclear about a previous history of chickenpox in childhood and visits her general practitioner.

What is the most appropriate next step?

a) Administer varicella-zoster immunoglobulin (VZIG)
b) Administer VZIG + varicella vaccine
c) Administer varicella vaccine
d) Reassure and discharge in the absence of a rash
e) Test her booking bloods for IgG antibodies to varicella

176

A woman presents at 36 weeks of gestation with a history of a previous caesarean section. Her previous baby was affected by early-onset group B *Streptococcus* (GBS). She is keen to deliver vaginally. She has been assessed by a consultant obstetrician and is suitable for a vaginal delivery. Her vaginal swab at 36 weeks is negative for GBS.

What mode of delivery is best suited for her, considering her history?

a) Elective caesarean section at 39 + 0 with antibiotic prophylaxis against GBS
b) Elective caesarean section at 39 + 0 with routine surgical antibiotic prophylaxis
c) Vaginal delivery with antibiotic prophylaxis against GBS in active labour
d) Vaginal delivery with routine measures and assessment of the baby for infection at birth
e) Vaginal delivery with routine measures, as the swab in this pregnancy is negative

177

A primigravid woman is in spontaneous labour at term with an effective epidural anaesthesia. She has been in the second stage of labour for three hours with regular contractions 4 in 10. The head is not palpable per abdomen. The last vaginal examination confirmed the cervix is fully dilated, vertex presenting, station at the spines and right occiput posterior (ROP) position. The cardiotocogram (CTG) is reassuring. She has now been actively pushing for two hours.

What would be your immediate course of action?

a) Allow another hour of pushing
b) Caesarean section, category 2
c) Direct traction forceps in theatre
d) Instrumental delivery with ventouse with an occipito-posterior (OP) cup in theatre
e) Instrumental delivery with silastic cup in delivery suite room

178

A woman who is para 5 has polyhydramnios and pre-eclampsia. She has previously had five normal vaginal deliveries. Her progress of labour has been good with an active phase of labour lasting six hours. Delivery is now imminent.

What is the most appropriate immediate postpartum management?

a) Misoprostol 1000 μg PR post delivery
b) Oxytocin infusion 40 units at 125 mL/h post delivery
c) Oxytocin infusion 40 units at 125 mL/h + misoprostol 1000 μg PR post delivery
d) Syntometrine IM post delivery
e) 10 IU oxytocin IM post delivery

179

Uterine perforation is a complication of uterine manipulation that can cause severe morbidity and even mortality.

Which of the following procedures is associated with the highest risk of uterine perforation?

a) Evacuation of retained products of conception (ERPC) for postpartum haemorrhage
b) Hysteroscopy following endometrial ablation
c) Hysteroscopy for postmenopausal bleeding
d) Surgical termination of pregnancy (STOP)
e) Uterine manipulation at laparoscopy

180

A woman has undergone genetic testing for BRCA1 and BRCA2 gene carriage and has been told she is a carrier for the BRCA1 gene, with a relative risk of developing ovarian cancer of 5. She asks you to explain relative risk to her.

Which one of the following best describes relative risk?

a) The difference in risk of a particular condition between those who are affected and those who are not
b) The number of people who must be treated to result in benefit to one person
c) The odds of an event happening in the affected group, expressed as a proportion of the odds of an event happening in the unaffected group
d) The rate of disease in the affected group divided by the rate of disease in the control group multiplied by the usual rate of the disease in the unaffected group
e) The rate of disease in the affected group divided by the rate of disease in the unaffected group

181

A 30-year-old woman is referred to your gynaecology clinic having had a forceps delivery complicated by a haematoma four months previously. She is complaining of pain in the vulval, perineal and perianal region.

Which of the following would *not* support your diagnosis of pudendal neuralgia?

a) Pain much worse in the seated position
b) Pain radiates to anterior part of thigh
c) Reduced awareness of defecation
d) Sexual dysfunction
e) Urinary hesitancy and frequency

182

A 72-year-old woman who is generally fit and well is referred to you by the surgeons. She has been admitted with left iliac fossa pain, and an ultrasound scan has suggested that gynaecological review is warranted. Her ultrasound scan shows a small anteverted uterus with an endometrial thickness of 3 mm. The left ovary shows no obvious mass, while the right ovary contains a 3.2 × 4.2 × 4.9 mm simple cyst. There is no free fluid seen. Her CA-125 is 16 IU/mL.

How would you manage this woman?

a) Laparoscopic bilateral salpingo-oophorectomy
b) Laparoscopic oophorectomy
c) Refer for discussion at the multidisciplinary team meetings
d) Repeat ultrasound in 4 months
e) Ultrasound-guided aspiration of cyst

183

During a vaginal repair, the assisting junior doctor asks about the different suture materials used. At that point, you are using polyglactin (Vicryl). You explain it is absorbable.

How long does it take to be absorbed?

a) 45–60 days
b) 60–90 days
c) 90–120 days
d) 120–180 days
e) 180–210 days

184

A medical student is attending colposcopy clinic with you, and asks you why the area you are looking at is called the transformation zone of the cervix.

Which of the following best describes the transformation zone of the cervix?

a) Glandular transformation of squamous epithelium
b) Metaplastic transformation of columnar to squamous epithelium
c) Pre-cancerous transformation of squamous epithelium
d) Transformation from columnar to transitional epithelium
e) Transformation from squamous to transitional epithelium

185

A woman who is about to undergo an assisted vaginal delivery needs a pudendal nerve block as she has inadequate analgesia.

What are the three branches of the pudendal nerve?

a) Inferior rectal nerve, perineal nerve, dorsal nerve of the clitoris
b) Inferior rectal nerve, superior rectal nerve, perineal nerve
c) Perineal nerve, dorsal nerve of the clitoris, ilioinguinal nerve
d) Perineal nerve, ilioinguinal nerve, inferior gluteal nerve
e) Perineal nerve, inferior rectal nerve, superior gluteal nerve

186

A woman who is taking the combined oral contraceptive has been prescribed antibiotics by her general practitioner (GP). She attends the emergency gynaecology unit concerned about any need for barrier contraception, as her GP did not mention this.

Which drug is most likely to cause contraceptive failure?

a) Ciprofloxacin
b) Clindamycin
c) Erythromycin
d) Nitrofurantoin
e) Rifampicin

187

A 24-year-old woman is referred to the gynaecology clinic with a history of acne, hirsuitism and oligomenorrhoea. When you review the blood results, the testosterone is 8 nmol/L (normal < 1.5 nmol/L).

Which one of the following conditions would *not* be associated with a raised serum testosterone of 8 nmol/L?

a) Androgen-secreting tumour of the adrenal
b) Androgen-secreting tumour of the ovary
c) Congenital adrenal hyperplasia
d) Cushing's syndrome
e) Polycystic ovary syndrome

188

A 34-year-old woman is 20 weeks in her first pregnancy. Her anomaly scan shows truncus arteriosus. She accepts your offer of amniocentesis.

Which investigation on amniotic fluid is most likely to identify the underlying cause?

a) Array comparative genomic hybridization (CGH)
b) Fluorescence in-situ hybridization (FISH) for 7q11 deletion (Williams syndrome)
c) G-banded karyotyping
d) Multiplex ligation-dependent probe amplification (MLPA) for subtelomeric rearrangements
e) Quantitative fluorescence polymerase chain reaction (QF-PCR) for common trisomies

189

A pregnant woman with a body mass index (BMI) of 35 undergoes oral glucose tolerance testing (OGTT) at 24 weeks of gestation. A standard 75 g OGTT is performed.

According to World Health Organization (WHO) criteria, what results confirm a diagnosis of gestational diabetes?

a) Fasting glucose of 5.8 mmol/L
b) One-hour glucose of 6.1 mmol/L
c) One-hour glucose of 7.8 mmol/L
d) Two-hour glucose of 7.6 mmol/L
e) Two-hour glucose of 7.9 mmol/L

190

Basic neonatal resuscitation is life-saving, training is simple and feasible, and the cost is low.

Neonatal resuscitation training packages for traditional birth attendants have been shown in both randomized and non-randomized trials to reduce perinatal and neonatal deaths by:

a) 0–20%
b) 20–40%
c) 40–60%
d) 60–80%
e) > 80%

191

A 26-year-old known HIV-positive woman on highly active antiretroviral therapy (HAART) presents at 38 + 3 weeks to the obstetric assessment unit with confirmed pre-labour spontaneous rupture of membranes. Review of her blood tests taken at 36 weeks of gestation reveals a CD4 count of 300 cells/picolitre and an undetectable viral load. Her first child was born by spontaneous vaginal delivery in the Democratic Republic of the Congo three years previously.

Following British HIV Association (BHIVA) guidance, what should her management plan be?

a) Admit for induction of labour
b) Allow 24 hours for the onset of spontaneous labour
c) Await the onset of spontaneous labour but perform caesarean section if not delivered within 12 hours
d) Deliver by caesarean section once a course of intramuscular steroids is complete
e) Deliver by caesarean section immediately

192

A 24-year-old primiparous woman with an uncomplicated monochorionic diamniotic twin pregnancy attends your antenatal clinic at 34 weeks of gestation requesting a plan regarding the timing of her delivery. On ultrasound scan, both babies are cephalic presentation.

What is the most appropriate advice?

a) Await spontaneous onset of labour
b) Elective caesarean section at 36 weeks of gestation following intramuscular steroid administration
c) Elective caesarean section at 39 weeks of gestation
d) Induction of labour at 36 weeks of gestation following intramuscular steroid administration
e) Induction of labour at 38 weeks of gestation

193

A 34-year-old woman had a total abdominal hysterectomy for chronic menorrhagia following unsuccessful endometrial ablation. Postoperatively, she complains of weakness of the left leg, along with paraesthesia over the anterior and medial thigh.

What is the most likely injury causing her symptoms?

a) Injury to femoral nerve
b) Injury to ilioinguinal and hypogastric nerves
c) Injury to lateral cutaneous nerve
d) Injury to obturator nerve
e) Injury to sciatic and common peroneal nerve

194

A 36-year-old woman was noted to have a blood pressure of 160/100 mmHg three days after a normal vaginal delivery at 38 weeks of gestation. She was offered induction of labour following diagnosis of pre-eclampsia at 37 weeks + 3 days. She is an asthmatic and uses inhalers. Her latest blood results are haemoglobin 105 g/L (normal 115–165), platelets 180 × 10^9/L (normal 150–400), creatinine 100 μmol/L (normal 53–97), alanine transaminase (ALT) 35 IU/L (normal 5–40). She is not breastfeeding.

What is the most appropriate antihypertensive for this woman?

a) Bendroflumethiazide
b) Labetalol
c) Methyldopa
d) Nifedepine
e) Ramipril

195

A 20-year-old woman presents to the emergency department with a short history of feeling unwell, fever and rigor two days after a vaginal delivery. Her pulse rate is 120 bpm, blood pressure 80/50 mmHg, temperature 38.5 °C, urine dipstick clear. An offensive lochia was noted on examination and vaginal swabs were taken. Full blood count revealed a white cell count of 23 × 10^9/L (normal 4–11), C-reactive protein 150 mg/L (normal < 10). An arterial blood gas showed lactate of 4 mmol/L (normal 0.5–2.2).

What should the next step in her investigation be?

a) Blood culture
b) Chest x-ray
c) Pelvic ultrasound
d) MRSA swabs
e) Urine culture

196

A 34-year-old woman with known HIV on highly active antiretroviral treatment (HAART) comes to the labour ward at 37 weeks of gestation with pre-labour spontaneous rupture of membranes. She had a plasma viral load of < 50 copies/mL at 36 weeks. She has no other obstetric complications.

What is the most appropriate mode of delivery?

a) Augmentation of labour at 24 hours
b) Await spontaneous labour
c) Caesarean section at 24 hours after steroid administration
d) Emergency caesarean section
e) Immediate augmentation of labour

197

A 25-year-old woman is seen on the postnatal ward complaining of feeling unwell with fever and rigors two days after a caesarean delivery. Her pulse rate is 120 bpm, blood pressure 80/50 mmHg, temperature 38.5 °C, urine dipstick clear. She is noted to have an offensive lochia. Investigations reveal a white cell count of 23 × 10^9/L (normal 4–11), C-reactive protein 150 mg/L (normal < 10). An arterial blood gas shows lactate of 4 mmol/L (normal 0.5–2.2). Examination of the scar reveals violet discoloration around the edges with small blisters.

What is the most likely infective organism?

a) Anaerobes
b) *Escherichia coli*
c) *Clostridium perfringens*
d) Group A *Streptococcus*
e) Group B *Streptococcus*

198

A 65-year-old woman presents with a sensation of a vaginal lump. She had a total abdominal hysterectomy for heavy periods 30 years ago. Examination reveals a vault prolapse.

On the POPQ scoring system, which point corresponds to the vaginal vault?

a) Aa
b) Bp
c) C
d) D
e) Tvl

199

A 30-year-old woman in her first pregnancy is admitted in labour at 36 weeks of gestation. Vaginal examination showed the cervix to be 6 cm dilated. The membranes ruptured soon after with blood-stained amniotic fluid. Following this, the fetal heart pattern changed and was interpreted as a sinusoidal trace.

What is the most appropriate management?

a) Augmentation with oxytocin
b) Caesarean section
c) Fetal blood sampling
d) Kleihauer test
e) Ultrasound with Doppler

200

A 34-year-old presented to the delivery suite with a history of a sudden gush of watery vaginal discharge. She is 30 weeks pregnant in her first pregnancy, which is uncomplicated. A vaginal speculum examination confirmed ruptured membranes with clear liquor draining. A scan confirmed cephalic presentation. She was asked to attend the day assessment clinic twice weekly.

Which investigation is most likely to identify chorioamnionitis?

a) Biophysical profile
b) Blood test for C-reactive protein
c) Cardiotocography
d) Full blood count
e) Vaginal swabs

Correct responses

Correct responses

1.	b	35.	c	69.	a
2.	b	36.	e	70.	c
3.	d	37.	c	71.	b
4.	b	38.	c	72.	c
5.	b	39.	b	73.	c
6.	c	40.	e	74.	b
7.	d	41.	a	75.	b
8.	b	42.	d	76.	c
9.	c	43.	c	77.	a
10.	e	44.	b	78.	e
11.	a	45.	d	79.	d
12.	e	46.	a	80.	a
13.	a	47.	d	81.	c
14.	d	48.	d	82.	c
15.	c	49.	b	83.	e
16.	b	50.	d	84.	b
17.	b	51.	c	85.	c
18.	e	52.	c	86.	c
19.	a	53.	b	87.	a
20.	a	54.	a	88.	a
21.	d	55.	a	89.	e
22.	e	56.	b	90.	d
23.	d	57.	e	91.	a
24.	b	58.	b	92.	c
25.	d	59.	b	93.	b
26.	b	60.	b	94.	b
27.	b	61.	d	95.	c
28.	a	62.	a	96.	c
29.	a	63.	a	97.	d
30.	c	64.	d	98.	e
31.	b	65.	c	99.	d
32.	c	66.	c	100.	a
33.	e	67.	d	101.	b
34.	b	68.	d	102.	c

Correct responses

103.	b	136.	c	169.	c
104.	c	137.	d	170.	e
105.	e	138.	c	171.	b
106.	e	139.	a	172.	c
107.	b	140.	a	173.	d
108.	c	141.	d	174.	d
109.	a	142.	a	175.	e
110.	b	143.	d	176.	c
111.	d	144.	e	177.	d
112.	a	145.	b	178.	e
113.	d	146.	c	179.	a
114.	d	147.	c	180.	e
115.	d	148.	b	181.	b
116.	c	149.	e	182.	d
117.	e	150.	e	183.	b
118.	e	151.	d	184.	b
119.	d	152.	c	185.	a
120.	c	153.	d	186.	e
121.	c	154.	e	187.	e
122.	d	155.	c	188.	a
123.	b	156.	b	189.	e
124.	d	157.	c	190.	b
125.	c	158.	c	191.	a
126.	d	159.	b	192.	d
127.	b	160.	e	193.	a
128.	d	161.	b	194.	d
129.	a	162.	e	195.	a
130.	b	163.	c	196.	e
131.	a	164.	a	197.	d
132.	d	165.	e	198.	c
133.	a	166.	b	199.	b
134.	a	167.	d	200.	c
135.	b	168.	d		

Explanations

Explanations

1

A 32-year-old woman attends her general practitioner surgery concerned that she has forgotten to take her oral contraceptive pills for the previous two days, having taken the first five tablets in the packet. She had unprotected sexual intercourse last night.

What is the most appropriate contraceptive advice?

a) Advise her to miss her forgotten pills and take her next pill at the usual time
b) Advise her that you recommend emergency contraception
c) Advise her to take her forgotten pills now and the next one at the usual time
d) Advise her to take her forgotten pills now and the next one at the usual time and start the next packet omitting the pill-free 7 days
e) Advise her to take her forgotten pills now and the next one at the usual time and use additional contraceptive for the next 7 days

Correct response: b

Explanation

Emergency contraception is recommended if two or more pills are missed from the first seven tablets in a packet and there has been unprotected sexual intercourse since finishing the last packet. A woman who has forgotten her combined oral contraceptive pill for less than 24 hours should be advised to take her forgotten pill now and the next one at the usual time. Additional contraception would only be required if she had missed two or more pills.

BNF. https://www.medicinescomplete.com/mc/bnf/current/PHP4869-combined-hormonal-contraceptives.htm (accessed 17 November 2014).
Faculty of Sexual & Reproductive Healthcare. *Clinical Guidance: Combined Hormonal Contraception*, August 2012. http://www.fsrh.org/pdfs/CEUGuidanceCombinedHormonalContraception.pdf (accessed 17 November 2014).

2

A community midwife booking a woman at 10 weeks of gestation is concerned that she might have had female genital mutilation (FGM). She speaks to the registrar, who enquires about the patient's country of origin.

Which country has the highest reported prevalence of FGM?

a) Nigeria
b) Somalia
c) Togo
d) Tanzania
e) Yemen

Correct response: b

Explanation
In Somalia the prevalence of FGM is 95–100%; in the other countries listed it is < 25%.

Royal College of Obstetricians & Gynaecologists. *Female Genital Mutilation and its Management*. Green-top Guideline No. 53, May 2009.

3

A 33-year-old woman has primary infertility due to bilateral hydrosalpinges. She has been referred for assisted reproduction. She is otherwise fit and well with no significant past medical history of note.

What initial treatment would optimize her chances of pregnancy with in-vitro fertilization (IVF)?

a) Aspiration of hydrosalpinx fluid
b) Hysteroscopic proximal tubal occlusion
c) Laparoscopic proximal tubal occlusion
d) Salpingectomy
e) Salpingostomy

Correct response: d

Explanation
The detrimental effect of hydrosalpinx on the outcome of IVF is now well documented, and a randomized controlled trial has reported a twofold increase in success rates with IVF after salpingectomy compared with no surgery. The role of other treatment options (proximal tubal occlusion, salpingostomy and aspiration of fluid) is unclear and needs to be evaluated further by large-scale research trials.

Suresh YN, Narvekar N. Role of surgery to optimise outcome of assisted conception treatments. *The Obstetrician & Gynaecologist* 2013; **15**: 91–8.

4

A 30-year-old woman had a vaginal delivery and also required manual removal of the placenta under spinal anaesthesia. She is known to be rhesus negative and her baby is confirmed to be rhesus positive. The Kleihauer test shows fetomaternal haemorrhage (FMH) of 5 mL.

How much anti-D should this woman receive?

a) 500 IU
b) 625 IU
c) 750 IU
d) 875 IU
e) 1000 IU

Correct response: b

Explanation

Studies have shown that approximately 99% of women have an FMH of less than 4 mL at delivery. Of the cases where the FMH is greater than 4 mL, 50% will have occurred during normal delivery. Manual removal of the placenta is one of the clinical circumstances that is more likely to be associated with a large FMH. In the UK, testing to quantify the size of FMH is recommended. An intramuscular dose of 500 IU of anti-D immunoglobulin will neutralize an FMH of up to 4 mL. For each millilitre of FMH in excess of 4 mL, a further 125 IU of anti-D immunoglobulin is necessary.

Royal College of Obstetricians & Gynaecologists. *The Use of Anti-D Immunoglobulin for Rhesus D Prophylaxis*. Green-top Guideline No. 52, March 2011.

5

You are a working as a fifth-year specialist trainee. A first-year specialist trainee asks you to observe her taking a history and performing an abdominal examination.

Which assessment tool is most appropriate to provide feedback on her history-taking skills?

a) CbD (case-based discussion)
b) Mini-CEX (mini clinical evaluation exercise)
c) OSATS (objective structured assessment of technical skill)
d) PQ (patient questionnaire)
e) TO1 (team observation)

Correct response: b

Explanation

The mini-CEX is used to assess history taking, examination and communication skills. The CbD assesses clinical reasoning. OSATS assesses technical skills during surgery. TO1 assesses attitude, professionalism and communication. The patient questionnaire is completed by the patient and assesses the doctor's attitude, professionalism and communication.

Shehmar M, Khan KS. A guide to the ATSM in Medical Education: Article 3: teaching and assessment in the clinical setting. *The Obstetrician & Gynaecologist* 2010; **12**: 199–205.

6

You have performed a hysterectomy on a 40-year-old woman for heavy menstrual bleeding. She has no significant medical history. Histology shows completely excised cervical intraepithelial neoplasia (CIN) grade 3. She is on routine recall for her smears and they have all been normal previously.

According to the NHS Cervical Screening Programme (NHSCSP) guidelines, when should she have vaginal vault cytology?

a) 3 and 6 months
b) 6 and 12 months
c) 6 and 18 months
d) 6, 12 and 18 months
e) 6, 12 and 24 months

Correct response: c

Explanation
Women who undergo hysterectomy and have completely excised CIN should have vaginal vault cytology at 6 and 18 months following their hysterectomy. Vault cytology is outside the routine screening programme and should be managed in a colposcopy setting.

NHS Cervical Screening Programme. *Colposcopy and Programme Management: Guidelines for the NHS Cervical Screening Programme*, 2nd edition. NHSCSP Publication No. 20, May 2010.

7

A couple, both aged 28, have been trying to conceive for over two years. They are both fit and well, with a normal body mass index (BMI), and are non-smokers. Following thorough investigation, they have been given a diagnosis of unexplained subfertility.

What treatment would NICE (the National Institute for Health and Care Excellence) recommend is offered to this couple?

a) Clomifene citrate
b) Intracytoplasmic sperm injection (ICSI)
c) Intrauterine insemination (IUI)
d) In-vitro fertilization (IVF)
e) Letrozole

Correct response: d

Explanation
Advise women with unexplained infertility who are having regular unprotected sexual intercourse to try to conceive for a total of two years (this can include up to one year before their fertility investigations) before IVF will be considered. Offer IVF treatment to women with unexplained infertility who have not conceived after two years (this can include up to one year before their fertility investigations) of regular unprotected sexual intercourse. Do not offer oral ovarian stimulation agents (such as clomifene citrate, anastrozole or letrozole) to women with unexplained infertility.

National Institute for Health and Care Excellence (NICE). *Fertility: Assessment and Treatment for People with Fertility Problems*. NICE Clinical Guideline CG156, February 2013.

8

A 41-year-old primigravida with a body mass index (BMI) of 31 attends the antenatal clinic at 10 weeks of gestation. Her father has type 2 diabetes. In this pregnancy, she will require aspirin 75 mg daily and will require screening for gestational diabetes with a glucose tolerance test (GTT).

At what gestation should she commence the aspirin and be screened for diabetes?

a) Aspirin from 12 weeks and GTT between 16 and 20 weeks
b) Aspirin from 12 weeks and GTT between 24 and 28 weeks
c) Aspirin from 16 weeks and GTT between 16 and 20 weeks
d) Aspirin from 16 weeks and GTT between 24 and 28 weeks
e) Aspirin from 16 weeks and GTT between 28 and 32 weeks

Correct response: b

Explanation
This woman has two risk factors for diabetes – her family history and her weight – but that does not mean she needs screening any earlier than recommended at 24–28 weeks. If she had had gestational diabetes in a previous pregnancy she should be screened at 16–18 weeks. She has more than one moderate risk factor – her age and first pregnancy – so needs aspirin from 12 weeks.

National Institute for Health and Care Excellence (NICE). *Diabetes in Pregnancy: Management of Diabetes and its Complications from Pre-Conception to the Postnatal Period*. NICE Clinical Guideline CG63, March 2008.

National Institute for Health and Care Excellence (NICE). *Hypertension in Pregnancy: the Management of Hypertensive Disorders during Pregnancy*. NICE Clinical Guideline CG107, August 2010.

9

A 35-year-old woman who has had two previous vaginal deliveries at 40 weeks has tested positive for HIV on antenatal screening. At booking, her viral load is reported as 150 copies/mL. She is otherwise well and is commenced on HAART (highly active antiretroviral therapy). At 36 weeks, her viral load is 75 copies/mL and there are no other obstetric complications.

What is the most appropriate delivery plan?

a) Await spontaneous labour
b) Caesarean section at 38 weeks
c) Caesarean section at 39 weeks
d) Induction of labour at 37 weeks
e) Induction of labour after 41 weeks

Correct response: c

Explanation
Vaginal delivery is recommended for women on HAART with a viral load < 50 HIV RNA copies/mL of plasma at gestational week 36. Above this level, elective caesarean section is recommended, since it is associated with an 80% decreased risk of mother-to-child transmission (MTCT).

British HIV Association guidelines for the management of HIV infection in pregnant women 2012. *HIV Medicine* 2012; **13** (Suppl. 2): 87–157. http://www.bhiva.org/documents/Guidelines/Pregnancy/2012/hiv1030_6.pdf (accessed 17 November 2014).

10

A 38-year-old primiparous woman attends for review following her 20-week scan. She has a history of systemic lupus erythematosus (SLE) diagnosed five years ago, predominantly causing joint and skin symptoms. On scan, the baby's heart was structurally normal with a rate of 80 bpm.

What is the most likely cause of the fetal heart rate of 80 bpm?

a) Anticardiolipin antibodies
b) Anti-double-stranded DNA
c) Anti-nuclear antibodies
d) Ribonuclear protein antibodies
e) Sjögren's syndrome A antibodies

Correct response: e

Explanation
The most likely diagnosis here is heart block secondary to autoimmune damage to the fetal heart, caused by Sjögren's syndrome A (SSA) antibodies or Sjögren's syndrome B (SSB) antibodies, previously called anti-Ro and anti-La.

Nelson-Piercy C. Autoimmune conditions. In Luesley DM, Baker PN, eds., *Obstetrics and Gynaecology: an Evidence-based Text for MRCOG*, 2nd edition. London: E. Arnold, 2010, pp. 92–7.

11

A 46-year-old woman had total abdominal hysterectomy for heavy menstrual bleeding due to a multiple fibroid uterus. Postoperatively, she had extreme difficulty in climbing the stairs. There is also some paraesthesia over the anterior and medial thigh as well as the medial aspect of the calf.

Which nerve has been injured during the operation?

a) Femoral nerve
b) Genitofemoral nerve
c) Ilioinguinal nerve
d) Obturator nerve
e) Sciatic nerve

Correct response: a

Explanation
In reports of gynaecological-associated neuropathy, the femoral nerve is most frequently injured, with an incidence of at least 11%. This happens when excessively deep retractor blades are used or during the lateral placement of retractors.

Kuponiyi O, Alleemudder DI, Latunde-Dada A, Eadarapalli P. Nerve injuries associated with gynaecological surgery. *The Obstetrician & Gynaecologist* 2014; **16**: 29–36.

12

A 21-year-old woman presents four days after unprotected sexual intercourse requesting emergency contraception. She is undergoing treatment for *Chlamydia*.

What is the most appropriate medication?

a) Levonorgestrel
b) Medroxyprogesterone acetate
c) Mifepristone
d) Norethisterone acetate
e) Ulipristal acetate

Correct response: e

Explanation
Ulipristal acetate and an intrauterine device (IUD) are licensed for use up to 120 hours after unprotected sexual intercourse or contraceptive failure.

Faculty of Sexual and Reproductive Healthcare. *Clinical Guidance: Emergency Contraception*, January 2012. http://www.fsrh.org/pdfs/CEUguidanceEmergencyContraception11.pdf (accessed 17 November 2014).

Murdoch M, Roberts M. Selective progesterone receptor modulators and their use within gynaecology. *The Obstetrician & Gynaecologist* 2014; **16**: 46–50.

13

A woman attends the antenatal clinic at 12 weeks of gestation requesting cervical cerclage as she has previously had a LLETZ (large loop excision of the transformation zone) for cervical dyskaryosis and is anxious she will deliver prematurely.

Under what circumstance would cervical cerclage be indicated?

a) At 20 weeks she has a cervical length of 23 mm on transvaginal ultrasound scan
b) She had a previous delivery at 33 weeks
c) She has previously had a miscarriage at 18 weeks of gestation
d) The pregnancy is a twin pregnancy
e) There is funnelling on transvaginal ultrasound scan at 23 weeks

Correct response: a

Explanation

a) A cervical length < 25 mm before 24/40 is an indication for cerclage.
b) This patient would be best managed with cervical length surveillance.
c) There is no significant risk reduction by cerclage with a history of one or two preterm births/late miscarriages. Risk is reduced with cervical cerclage after a history of three preterm births/late miscarriages.
d) Multiple pregnancy is a contraindication to cerclage.
e) Funnelling in the absence of a shortened cervix is not an indication for cerclage.

Royal College of Obstetricians & Gynaecologists. *Cervical Cerclage*. Green-top Guideline No. 60, May 2011.

14

A woman with a body mass index (BMI) of 63 has a complicated labour and delivery and nearly dies.

Which of the following causes of maternal mortality is independent of her BMI?

a) Amniotic fluid embolism
b) Anaesthetic complications
c) Pre-eclampsia
d) Sepsis
e) Venous thromboembolism

Correct response: d

Explanation

Although maternal mortality and morbidity are increased with obesity and in general get worse the more obese the woman is, this does not hold for severe sepsis. In the UK Obstetric Surveillance System (UKOSS) study, quoted in *Saving mothers' lives*, the major risk factors for severe maternal sepsis were varied. The most important (adjusted odds ratio (aOR) 12.07, 95% confidence interval (CI) 8.11–17.97) was a febrile illness or taking antibiotics in the two weeks prior to presentation. Caesarean section after labour onset (aOR 8.06, 95% CI 4.65–13.97) was worse than pre-labour caesarean (aOR 3.83, 95% CI 2.24–6.56) or operative vaginal delivery (aOR 2.49, 95% CI 1.32–4.70).

Centre for Maternal and Child Enquiries (CMACE). Saving mothers' lives: reviewing maternal deaths to make motherhood safer: 2006–2008. The Eighth Report of the Confidential Enquiries into Maternal Deaths in the United Kingdom. *BJOG* 2011; 118 (Suppl. 1): 1–203.

15

You review a woman who is currently 30 weeks pregnant in her second pregnancy. She had deep venous thrombosis (DVT) in her last pregnancy. In her current pregnancy, she was commenced on prophylactic low-molecular-weight heparin (LMWH) once a day.

Compared to unfractionated heparin, which of the following statements about LMWH is most accurate?

a) LMWH binds more effectively to antithrombin III and enhances the inhibition of coagulation factor IXa
b) LMWH binds more strongly to endothelial cells and platelets
c) LMWH has a higher bioavailability at lower dose when administered subcutaneously
d) LMWH has a similar effect on bones and can induce osteoporosis
e) LMWH has a similar half life

Correct response: c

Explanation
A Cochrane review on prophylaxis for venous thromboembolic disease in pregnancy and the early postnatal period found that LMWH was more effective in preventing thrombosis than unfractionated heparin.

Bain E, Wilson A, Tooher R, *et al.* Prophylaxis for venous thromboembolic disease in pregnancy and the early postnatal period. *Cochrane Database of Systematic Reviews* 2014; (2): CD001689.
Royal College of Obstetricians & Gynaecologists. *Reducing the Risk of Thrombosis and Embolism during Pregnancy and the Puerperium*. Green-top Guideline No. 37a, November 2009.

16

A general practitioner has referred a 36-year-old woman to gynaecology outpatients because of her symptoms of intermenstrual bleeding as well as subfertility. Her pelvic scan is as follows:

Anteverted uterus measures 77 × 50 × 42 mm.
Myometrial appearances are suggestive of adenomyosis.
Endometrial thickness is 7 mm with a 10 × 15 mm mass at the fundus: ?polyp.
Both ovaries appear normal, with a 13 mm follicle in the left ovary.
No free fluid or adnexal masses seen.
She enquires about other investigations to confirm the presence of an endometrial polyp.

Which of the following modalities is considered to be the gold standard for diagnosing endometrial polyps?

a) CT scan of pelvis
b) Hysteroscopy
c) Pelvic ultrasound

d) Saline infusion sonogram
e) Transvaginal ultrasound

Correct response: b

Explanation
Saline infusion sonogram is more accurate than transvaginal ultrasound, but hysteroscopy allows treatment at the same time.

Annan JJ, Aquilina J, Ball E. The management of endometrial polyps in the 21st century. *The Obstetrician & Gynaecologist* 2012; **14**: 33–8.

17

A 46-year-old woman presents for assessment prior to a planned admission for abdominal hysterectomy. She has well-controlled type 2 diabetes and her body mass index (BMI) is 42. Her mother had a pulmonary embolism after hip replacement, but she was investigated and found to be negative for thrombophilia. The indication for hysterectomy is menorrhagia and anaemia caused by a large fibroid uterus. Her preoperative haemoglobin is 122 g/L.

What is the most important factor influencing a plan for anticoagulant prophylaxis?

a) Her age
b) Her BMI
c) Her family history of thrombosis
d) Her fibroid uterus
e) Her history of anaemia

Correct response: b

Explanation
Age and a fibroid uterus have no material impact on her risk of thrombosis. The anaemia has been corrected and the family history investigated previously. Her raised BMI is a significant risk factor for thrombosis and should prompt consideration of prophylaxis.

National Institute for Health and Care Excellence (NICE). *Venous Thromboembolism: Reducing the Risk.* NICE Clinical Guideline CG92, January 2010.

18

A 25-year-old para 1 woman sustained a 3a perineal tear following an instrumental delivery. She attends her postnatal follow-up appointment. She has no faecal incontinence, has no incontinence of flatus and the perineum has healed well.

What advice would you offer this woman with regard to subsequent delivery?

a) Avoiding prolonged second stage eliminates the risk of a third-degree tear
b) Early epidural reduces the risk of a third-degree tear
c) Elective caesarean section eliminates the risk of faecal incontinence in later life
d) Prophylactic episiotomy reduces the risk of a third-degree tear
e) Subsequent vaginal delivery is associated with a small additional risk of developing faecal incontinence

Correct response: e

Explanation

Between 60% and 80% of women will have no symptoms following a third-degree tear at 12 months. The commonest symptoms are incontinence of flatus and faecal urgency. Only around 11% will have faecal leakage. However, endoanal ultrasound in recent randomized control trials reveals defects in up to 36% of women, which may be why faecal incontinence can develop in later life.

Royal College of Obstetricians & Gynaecologists. *The Management of Third- and Fourth-degree Perineal Tears*. Green-top Guideline No. 29, March 2007.

19

A 32-year-old woman is brought into the emergency department with a one-day history of fever, rigors, abdominal pain and heavy lochia. She had an uncomplicated spontaneous vaginal delivery two days ago. On arrival, she has a temperature of 39 °C, a heart rate of 143 bpm, a blood pressure of 82/50 mmHg and a respiratory rate of 40/min.

Following initial resuscitation, what is the most appropriate immediate management?

a) Blood cultures and vaginal swabs
b) Broad-spectrum IV antibiotics
c) Evacuation of retained products of conception
d) IV dopamine
e) IV immunoglobulin

Correct response: a

Explanation

It is essential that blood cultures are taken initially, but IV antibiotics should be started immediately without waiting for culture. However, if the woman does not respond to initial antibiotics the cultures will be available to guide the clinical team. Antibiotics should be chosen to cover the common causes of puerperal sepsis, which are group A *Streptococcus* (GAS), *Escherichia coli*, *Staphylococcus aureus* and *Streptococcus pneumoniae*.

Royal College of Obstetricians & Gynaecologists. *Bacterial Sepsis Following Pregnancy*. Green-top Guideline No. 64b, April 2012.

20

A 45-year-old woman underwent a total abdominal hysterectomy for heavy menstrual bleeding. In the postoperative period she develops weakness of hip flexion and adduction and is unable to extend the knee. On examination the knee jerk reflex is lost and there is altered sensation over the medial aspect of thigh and calf.

What nerve is most likely to have been damaged?

a) Femoral nerve
b) Genitofemoral nerve
c) Ilioinguinal nerve
d) Obturator nerve
e) Pudendal nerve

Correct response: a

Explanation

Femoral neuropathy commonly occurs as a result of compression of the nerve against the pelvic sidewall as it emerges from the lateral border of the psoas muscle. This can occur when a self-retaining retractor with a deep blade is used during a hysterectomy.

Kuponiyi O, Alleemudder DI, Latunde-Dada A, Eadarapalli P. Nerve injuries associated with gynaecological surgery. *The Obstetrician & Gynaecologist* 2014; **16**: 29–36.

21

A primigravid woman attends the antenatal clinic with a query. She is a teacher and is 16 weeks pregnant and has been exposed to a student with slapped cheek syndrome about four weeks ago. As far as she is aware, she has never had this herself and is concerned about her pregnancy. A blood test is negative for IgG and positive for maternal IgM antibodies for parvovirus. An ultrasound scan reveals a normal viable pregnancy.

What advice would you give this woman regarding follow-up?

a) She can be reassured and discharged if a second scan in 4 weeks' time is normal
b) She can be reassured and discharged in view of the normal scan
c) She should have 4-weekly growth scans from 28 weeks
d) She should have fortnightly ultrasound scans until 30 weeks. If the scans are normal she can be reassured and discharged
e) She should have fortnightly ultrasound scans until delivery

Correct response: d

Explanation

The incubation period of parvovirus is 13–18 days and the person is infectious for 10 days prior to the appearance of the rash. Transplacental transmission occurs in a third of cases. In the second trimester, haematopoiesis occurs in the fetal liver and, because of the increased demand from the growing fetus, there is a 34-fold increase in red blood cell mass, concomitant with a reduction in red blood cell lifespan to 45–70 days. Because the virus attacks erythroid precursors, this leads to severe anaemia and high-output cardiac failure, often with added viral myocarditis, which leads to fetal hydrops. In the third trimester there is a larger blood volume and longer red cell lifespan, so less effect on the fetus.

Health Protection Agency. Guidance on viral rash in pregnancy, January 2011. http://www.hpa.org.uk/webc/HPAwebFile/HPAweb_C/1294740918985 (accessed 17 November 2014).
Lamont RF, Sobel JD, Vaisbuch E, *et al*. Parvovirus B19 infection in human pregnancy. *BJOG* 2011; **118**: 175–86.

22

Following the effective management of a shoulder dystocia, a first-year trainee approaches you to learn how to perform the manoeuvres to manage shoulder dystocia.

What is the most effective way of achieving this learning?

a) Attending a lecture
b) Brainstorming

c) Case-based discussion
d) Electronic learning
e) Simulation training

Correct response: e

Explanation
Simulation refers to the replacement or amplification of real experiences with ones that evoke or replicate substantial aspects of the real world in a fully interactive manner. It is useful for clinical and practical education, particularly for introducing new skills.

Crofts JF, Bartlett C, Ellis D, *et al*. Training for shoulder dystocia: a trial of simulation using low-fidelity and high-fidelity mannequins. *Obstetrics and Gynecology* 2006; **108**: 1477–85.

Royal College of Obstetricians & Gynaecologists. StratOG eLearning. https://stratog.rcog.org.uk (accessed 17 November 2014).

23

A primiparous woman presents two days after a normal vaginal delivery complaining of feeling unwell. On examination, she has a temperature of 38 °C, pulse rate of 110 bpm and blood pressure of 90/50 mmHg. There are no localizing signs of infection. Blood tests are performed.

What test result would indicate a severe sepsis?

a) C-reactive protein 53 mg/L (normal < 10)
b) Plasma glucose 12.2 mmol/L (normal 3.6–6.1)
c) Serum creatinine 90 mmol/L (normal 53–97)
d) Serum lactate 5 mmol/L (normal 0.5–2.2)
e) White cell count 13.1×10^9/L (normal $4–11 \times 10^9$)

Correct response: d

Explanation
'Red flag' signs and symptoms include pyrexia > 38 °C, a sustained tachycardia and a respiratory rate > 20 breaths/minute. Blood cultures are key investigations prior to IV antibiotics. Lactate should be measured within six hours of the suspicion of severe sepsis, since a level of 4 mmol/L or more is indicative of tissue hypoperfusion.

Royal College of Obstetricians & Gynaecologists. *Bacterial Sepsis Following Pregnancy*. Green-top Guideline No. 64b, April 2012.

24

A 59-year-old para 2 woman presents with postmenopausal bleeding. She is found to have an endometrial thickness of 11 mm on ultrasound scan and is booked for an outpatient hysteroscopy.

What is the ideal size of hysteroscope for her procedure?

a) 2.2 mm hysteroscope with 2.5–3 mm sheath
b) 2.7 mm hysteroscope with 3–3.5 mm sheath
c) 2.7 mm hysteroscope with 4–5 mm sheath

d) 3 mm hysteroscope with 3.5–4 mm sheath
e) 3 mm hysteroscope with 4.5–5 mm sheath

Correct response: b

Explanation
Although flexible hysteroscopes are associated with less pain, the images are poorer, there is a greater chance of a failed procedure, it takes longer to perform and the overall costs are higher.

Royal College of Obstetricians & Gynaecologists. *Best Practice in Outpatient Hysteroscopy*. Green-top Guideline No. 59, March 2011.

25

A 25-year-old woman has been having persistently high blood pressure of > 150/100 mmHg for three days following delivery with no biochemical or haematological abnormalities. She has no underlying medical problems and was not on any antihypertensive drugs during the pregnancy. She is breastfeeding.

Which is the most appropriate antihypertensive agent that can be prescribed for her?

a) Amlodipine
b) Bendroflumethiazide
c) Candesartan
d) Enalapril
e) Methyldopa

Correct response: d

Explanation
Enalapril and captopril have no adverse effects on babies who are breastfeeding. There is insufficient evidence for other ACE inhibitors. A beta-blocker would have been an alternative answer, but there is none in the option list.

National Institute for Health and Care Excellence (NICE). *Hypertension in Pregnancy: the Management of Hypertensive Disorders during Pregnancy*. NICE Clinical Guideline CG107, August 2010.
Smith M, Waugh J, Nelson-Piercy C. Management of postpartum hypertension. *The Obstetrician & Gynaecologist* 2013; **15**: 45–50.

26

In the Confidential Enquiry into Maternal Deaths, sepsis was the leading cause of maternal mortality in the UK between 2006 and 2008.

Which one of the following most accurately represents the mortality rate of severe sepsis with acute organ dysfunction?

a) 1–10%
b) 21–30%
c) 41–50%
d) 61–70%
e) 81–90%

Correct response: b

Explanation
The mortality rate related to sepsis increased from 0.85 deaths per 100 000 maternities in 2003–05 to 1.13 deaths in 2006–08, and sepsis was the most common cause of direct maternal death in the latest report. Delay in recognizing the severity of the infection and delay in starting antibiotics were significant learning points. It was also commented that inadequate doses and oral therapy were identified as factors, noting that aggressive treatment in the first 'golden hour' offers the best chance of recovery.

Centre for Maternal and Child Enquiries (CMACE). Saving mothers' lives: reviewing maternal deaths to make motherhood safer: 2006–2008. The Eighth Report of the Confidential Enquiries into Maternal Deaths in the United Kingdom. *BJOG* 2011; 118 (Suppl. 1): 1–203.

Royal College of Obstetricians & Gynaecologists. *Bacterial Sepsis in Pregnancy*. Green-top Guideline No. 64a, April 2012.

27

You are about to repair a second-degree tear under local anaesthetic in a woman with no previous analgesia. Her most recent weight in pregnancy was 50 kg.

What is the maximum volume of 1% lidocaine (when not mixed with adrenaline) that can be used?

a) 10 mL
b) 15 mL
c) 20 mL
d) 25 mL
e) 30 mL

Correct response: b

Explanation
3 mg/kg of plain 1% (10 mg/mL) lidocaine (previously known as lignocaine) is the maximum dose before toxicity. Signs of toxicity usually start 1–5 minutes after injection but may be delayed up to an hour. The classical symptoms are related to the central nervous system and include numbness of the tongue or around the mouth, a metallic taste in the mouth, dizziness or feeling light-headed, and they can include disorientation, drowsiness, tinnitus or problems focusing.

Anaesthesia UK. Pharmacology of regional anaesthesia. http://www.frca.co.uk/article.aspx?articleid=100816 (accessed 17 November 2014).

28

An ST6 doctor (postgraduate doctor in year 6 of specialty training) attends an appraisal meeting with her educational supervisor.

Which one of the following statements best describes the appraisal process?

a) Personal and educational development are discussed with agreed goals
b) The educational supervisor provides an assessment and review of performance
c) The educational supervisor provides the trainee with objective evidence of her progress

d) The educational supervisor reviews progress and recommends the educational targets to be achieved
e) This is a summative assessment of the trainee's progress

Correct response: a

Explanation
Different methods of assessment are used to support training.

Shehmar M, Khan KS. A guide to the ATSM in Medical Education. Article 2: assessment, feedback and evaluation. *The Obstetrician & Gynaecologist* 2010; **12**: 119–25.

29

A medical student is interested in learning about enhanced recovery in gynaecology.

Which of the following principles is *not* part of an enhanced recovery pathway?

a) Antibiotic prophylaxis following the skin incision
b) Avoidance of intraoperative hypothermia
c) Complex carbohydrate drinks 4 hours prior to surgery
d) Early postoperative feeding
e) Verbal and written information for the patient explaining the perioperative pathway

Correct response: a

Explanation
Enhanced recovery aims to speed up a patient's recovery from theatre, improving outcomes. By preparing the patient beforehand, optimizing intraoperative and postoperative management and thus reducing stress, and mobilizing the patient early, complications are reduced and recovery improved.

NHS Institute for Improvement and Innovation. Enhanced recovery programme. http://www.institute.nhs.uk/quality_and_service_improvement_tools/quality_and_service_improvement_tools/enhanced_recovery_programme.html (accessed 17 November 2014).
Torbé E, Crawford R, Nordin A, Acheson N. Enhanced recovery in gynaecology. *The Obstetrician & Gynaecologist* 2013; **15**: 263–8.

30

You have just completed the last case on the afternoon theatre list, having assisted with a hysterectomy with your consultant, and she requests you to complete the WHO sign-out while she finishes writing up the operating notes.

Which of the following is *not* usually part of a WHO surgical sign-out?

a) Has it been confirmed that instruments, swabs and sharps counts are complete?
b) Has the name of the procedure been recorded?
c) Has the scheduling of the list workload been appropriate?
d) Have any equipment problems been identified that need to be addressed?
e) Have the specimens been labelled (including patient name)?

Correct response: c

Explanation
Surgery is intended to save lives and suffering, but at times it will cause damage to the patient. Complications from surgery occur in up to 25% of cases, and in many situations this is considered preventable. The World Health Organization (WHO) surgical safety checklist is used throughout the world to help prevent avoidable surgical mishaps.

World Health Organization. *WHO Guidelines for Safe Surgery 2009: Safe Surgery Saves Lives*. Geneva: WHO, 2009.

31

The cardiovascular system undergoes immense physiological changes in pregnancy.

Which of the following parameters does *not* change in pregnancy?

a) Cardiac output
b) Central venous pressure
c) Heart rate
d) Stroke volume
e) Systemic vascular resistance

Correct response: b

Explanation
Cardiac output increases early in pregnancy. The blood volume rises from five weeks after conception, which, coupled with a reduction in systemic vascular resistance secondary to oestrogen and prostaglandins, leads to the increased cardiac output. The increased cardiac output is achieved by an increase in stroke volume and also a rise in the heart rate.

Nelson-Piercy C. *Handbook of Obstetric Medicine*, 4th edition. London: Informa Healthcare, 2010.

32

There are huge changes in the coagulation system in pregnancy.

Which of the following components of the coagulation system does *not* change in an uncomplicated pregnancy?

a) Factor IX
b) Fibrinogen
c) Platelets
d) Protein S
e) Von Willebrand's factor

Correct response: c

Explanation
Venous thromboembolism (VTE) is up to 10 times more common in pregnancy than in the non-pregnant population. This is due to the increase in many clotting factors, a decrease in protein S and a reduction in fibrinolysis. There is also a reduction in venous blood flow during pregnancy, especially in the left femoral vein, and the risk of pelvic venous trauma during delivery, especially if instrumental.

Edmonds DK. *Dewhurst's Textbook of Obstetrics and Gynaecology*, 8th edition. Chichester: Wiley, 2012.

Nelson-Piercy C. *Handbook of Obstetric Medicine*, 4th edition. London: Informa Healthcare, 2010.

33

In the most recent Confidential Enquiry into Maternal Deaths (2006–08), sepsis was the leading cause of direct maternal deaths.

Among the direct maternal deaths due to sepsis, which were the most common risk factors to predict those who died?

a) Body mass index (BMI) 40+, over 40 years, primiparity
b) BMI 40+, under 40 years, multiparity
c) BMI 40+, under 40 years, primiparity
d) Normal BMI, under 40 years, primiparity
e) Normal BMI, under 40 years, multiparity

Correct response: e

Explanation

Although obesity is a factor in many complications of pregnancy, deaths due to sepsis were more common in women who appeared to be at lower risk.

Centre for Maternal and Child Enquiries (CMACE). Saving mothers' lives: reviewing maternal deaths to make motherhood safer: 2006–2008. The Eighth Report of the Confidential Enquiries into Maternal Deaths in the United Kingdom. *BJOG* 2011; **118** (Suppl. 1): 1–203.

34

A 23-year-old primigravid woman presents at the emergency department at six weeks of gestation with threatened miscarriage. On examination, her vital signs are normal and abdomen is soft and there is minimal tenderness on deep palpation. On speculum examination, there is a small amount of brown (old) blood in the vagina. A transvaginal ultrasound scan shows an intrauterine gestation sac, measuring 38 × 25 × 20 mm. A yolk sac is visible, and a fetal pole is visible measuring 6 mm. No fetal heart activity is seen. A small area of subchorionic haemorrhage is seen.

What would be the best management plan for her?

a) Arrange for a dating scan at 12 weeks
b) Arrange for a repeat scan after 7 days
c) Arrange for a serial serum beta-hCG level
d) Arrange for a serum progesterone level
e) Arrange surgical management of miscarriage

Correct response: b

Explanation

In an early pregnancy with crown–rump length (CRL) < 7 mm and no fetal heart activity, a second scan should be performed at a minimum of seven days after the first before making a diagnosis of miscarriage. Once a gestation sac has been identified, there is no role for serum human chorionic gonadotrophin (hCG) or serum progesterone level.

National Institute for Health and Care Excellence (NICE). *Ectopic Pregnancy and Miscarriage: Diagnosis and Initial Management in Early Pregnancy of Ectopic Pregnancy and Miscarriage*. NICE Clinical Guideline CG154, December 2012.

35

A 35-year-old primigravida is referred to the antenatal clinic at 32 weeks of gestation. The midwife performed a blood test to check her liver function tests a week ago when she had an itchy rash. The rash has disappeared and she is no longer itchy. Her blood pressure is 110/70 mmHg and there is no proteinuria. Examination is normal. The results show:

Total bilirubin 7 µmol/L (normal 0–17)
Alkaline phosphatase 183 IU/L (normal 30–130)
Alanine transaminase 28 IU/L (normal 0–40)
Albumin 32 g/L (normal 35–46)

What is the most appropriate blood test?

a) Check prothrombin time
b) Check serum total bile acids
c) No blood test required
d) Repeat liver function tests
e) Test for viral hepatitis

Correct response: c

Explanation
Alkaline phosphatase may increase up to 3× normal during pregnancy due to placental isoenzymes. Albumin is reduced with haemodilution. With normal liver function tests and the resolution of symptoms, no further tests are required.

Walker I, Chappell LC, Williamson C. Abnormal liver function tests in pregnancy. *BMJ* 2013; **347**: f6055.

36

A 28-year-old nulliparous woman has had two consecutive miscarriages in the first trimester. She is referred with a further non-viable pregnancy at eight weeks of gestation.

What is the most appropriate genetic test to perform?

a) Karyotype both partners
b) Karyotype chorionic villus sample in next pregnancy
c) Karyotype father
d) Karyotype mother
e) Karyotype products of conception

Correct response: e

Explanation
Karyotyping the parents is no longer considered appropriate unless there is an abnormality found within products of conception. Tissue should be sent from the products of conception of a third miscarriage.

Royal College of Obstetricians & Gynaecologists. *The Investigation and Treatment of Couples with Recurrent First-trimester and Second-trimester Miscarriage*. Green-top Guideline No. 17, April 2011.

37

A nulliparous woman presents with lower abdominal pain in early pregnancy. The human chorionic gonadotrophin (hCG) level is 986 IU/L. At laparoscopy the following is found:

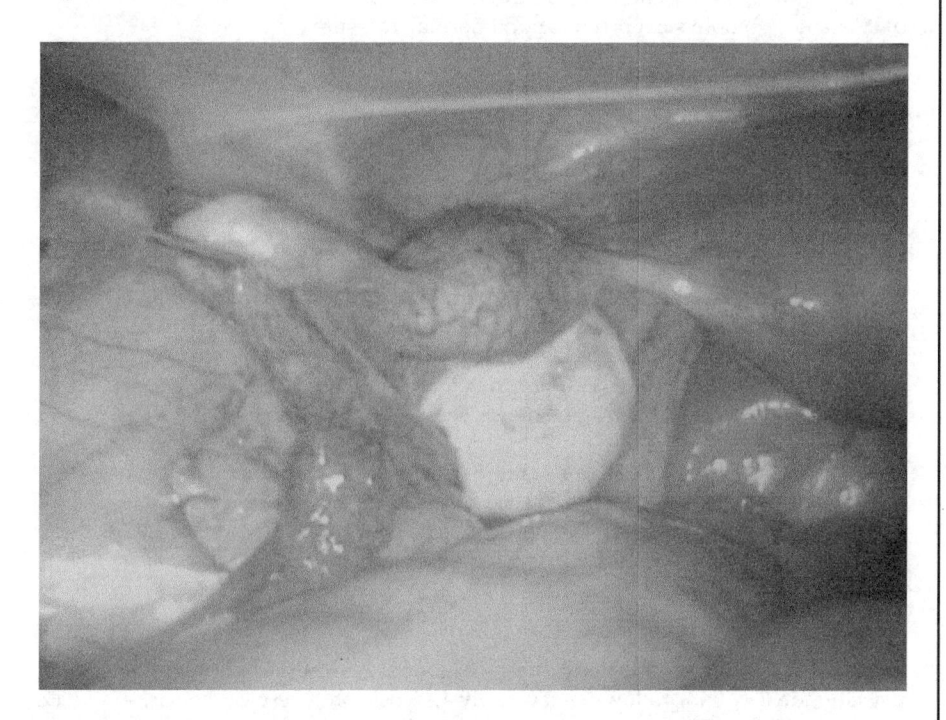

There is no other abnormality seen in the pelvis.

What is the most appropriate management option?

a) Inject methotrexate into mass
b) Intramuscular methotrexate injection
c) Left salpingectomy
d) Left salpingo-oophorectomy
e) Left salpingostomy

Correct response: c

Explanation

If the other tube looks normal, salpingectomy should be performed. There is no increase in intrauterine pregnancies, and the risk of ectopic pregnancy is higher, with salpingostomy. If salpingostomy is performed, follow-up is essential to identify those women with persistent trophoblast.

Royal College of Obstetricians & Gynaecologists. *The Management of Tubal Pregnancy*. Green-top Guideline No. 21, May 2004, reviewed 2010.

38

A 34-year-old primigravida presents to the maternity assessment unit with a second episode of decreased fetal movements at 38 + 4 weeks of gestation. She is known to be low risk and has had an otherwise uneventful pregnancy. An ultrasound scan a week ago was normal, with the baby on the 50th centile.

What is the most appropriate management option?

a) Advise formal kick counting and review in 2 days
b) Arrange a biophysical profile and, if normal, reassure
c) Consider induction of labour
d) Perform cardiotocography (CTG) and arrange a further scan
e) Perform a CTG and, if normal, reassure

Correct response: c

Explanation

Women should be counselled in the antenatal period about the significance of fetal movement and its relation to stillbirths. There is no evidence that any formal definition of reduced fetal movement is of greater value than subjective maternal perception in the detection of fetal compromise. Biophysical profiling has not been shown to be of benefit. Induction of pregnancy may be appropriate following discussion with a senior obstetrician. The advantages and disadvantages should be discussed with the woman.

Unterscheider J, Horgan R, O'Donoghue K, Greene R. Reduced fetal movements. *The Obstetrician & Gynaecologist* 2009; **11**: 245–51.

Royal College of Obstetricians & Gynaecologists. *Reduced Fetal Movements*. Green-top Guideline No. 57, February 2011.

39

A 52-year-old woman has recently been diagnosed with cervical intraepithelial neoplasia grade 3 (CIN3) following severe dyskaryosis on a cervical smear. A LLETZ specimen shows CIN3 incompletely excised at the endocervical margin.

What is the most appropriate next step in her management?

a) Colposcopy and smear in 6 months
b) Loop excision immediately
c) Loop excision in 6 months
d) Smear in 6 months
e) Smear and high-risk human papillomavirus (HR-HPV) DNA testing in 6 months

Correct response: b

Explanation

In a series of 3426 LLETZ (large loop excision of the transformation zone) procedures, women older than 50 years with CIN at the margin of excision constituted a minor high-risk group. It was suggested that these women should be offered retreatment rather than surveillance.

NHS Cervical Screening Programme. *Colposcopy and Programme Management: Guidelines for the NHS Cervical Screening Programme*, 2nd edition. NHSCSP Publication No. 20, May 2010.

40

A 32-year-old woman with dull lower abdominal pain and bloating had a pelvic ultrasound scan arranged by her general practitioner. The results show a simple 30 mm right-sided ovarian cyst. There are no other concerns.

What is the most appropriate next step in her management?

a) Arrange for a repeat scan in 4 months
b) Arrange for a repeat scan in a year
c) Arrange further imaging with MRI/CT
d) Check serum CA-125
e) Reassure and discharge without follow-up

Correct response: e

Explanation

Premenopausal women with simple cysts less than 50 mm do not require follow-up, as these cysts are physiological and almost always resolve within three menstrual cycles.

Royal College of Obstetricians & Gynaecologists. *Management of Suspected Ovarian Masses in Premenopausal Women*. Green-top Guideline No. 62, November 2011.

41

A 34-year-old primigravid woman attends for her booking scan at 12 weeks of gestation. The report shows a live twin pregnancy with T sign present on ultrasound scan. The crown–rump length is equivalent to 12 + 5 for both twins.

What would you document in her plan of care?

a) Aim for delivery at 36–37 weeks
b) Caesarean section is the recommended mode of delivery
c) Quad test screening at 16 weeks
d) Refer to fetal medicine unit
e) Serial scan every 4 weeks

Correct response: a

Explanation

The T sign is seen in monochorionic twins, because there is no gap between the two amniotic sacs. The lambda sign occurs in dichorionic twins, as the two amniotic membranes meet the chorionic plate. This is best seen in early pregnancy and may not be able to be visualized later on. In this case, the woman should be treated as if the pregnancy is monochorionic.

Royal College of Obstetricians & Gynaecologists. *Management of Monochorionic Twin Pregnancy*. Green-top Guideline No. 51, December 2008.

42

A 37-year-old woman is due to have a diagnostic laparoscopy to investigate chronic pelvic pain. The overall risk of serious complications is 1 in 500.

What is the most appropriate way to explain this risk verbally?

a) Common
b) Rare
c) Unusual
d) Uncommon
e) Very rare

Correct response: d

Explanation

Percentages are an abstract way of portraying risk, whereas the actual number of people who could be affected is more vivid. Instead of saying 5%, say 5 out of 100 people or 1 in 20.

Uncommon	1/100 to 1/1000	A person in a village
Rare	1/1000 to 1/10 000	A person in a small town
Very rare	Less than 1/10 000	A person in a large town

Royal College of Obstetricians & Gynaecologists. *Presenting Information on Risk*. Clinical Governance Advice No. 7, December 2008.

43

A 54-year-old woman was referred to the outpatient hysteroscopy clinic with a history of a single episode of vaginal bleeding, which lasted for a day. She had her last period two years ago. A transvaginal ultrasound scan showed an endometrial thickness of 6 mm. She is nulliparous and her body mass index (BMI) is 47. She is very anxious and is requesting pain relief.

What is the most appropriate option for pain relief?

a) Codeine tablets orally about an hour before the procedure
b) Conscious sedation
c) Infiltration of local anaesthetic into the cervix
d) Instillation of local anaesthetic into the cervical canal
e) Not suitable for outpatient procedure; list under general anaesthesia

Correct response: c

Explanation

Instillation of local anaesthetic into the cervical canal does not reduce pain during diagnostic outpatient hysteroscopy but may reduce the incidence of vasovagal reactions. Topical application of local anaesthetic to the ectocervix should be considered where use of a cervical tenaculum is necessary. Application of local anaesthetic into or around the cervix is associated with a reduction in the pain experienced during outpatient diagnostic hysteroscopy. Consideration should be given to the routine administration of intracervical or paracervical local anaesthetic, particularly in postmenopausal women.

Conscious sedation should not be routinely used in outpatient hysteroscopic procedures, as it confers no advantage over local anaesthesia in terms of pain control and the woman's satisfaction. Routine use of opioid analgesia before outpatient hysteroscopy should be avoided, as it may cause adverse effects

Royal College of Obstetricians & Gynaecologists. *Best Practice in Outpatient Hysteroscopy*. Green-top Guideline No. 59, March 2011.

44

A woman who is 12 weeks pregnant has a first-trimester screening for Down's syndrome, which shows a high-risk result. The woman undergoes amniocentesis at 15 weeks of gestation.

What is the additional risk of miscarriage following amniocentesis?

a) 0.5%
b) 1%

c) 2%
d) 2.5%
e) 3%

Correct response: b

Explanation
Amniocentesis involves an increased risk of miscarriage, due to its invasive nature. The woman should be fully counselled regarding this risk.

Royal College of Obstetricians & Gynaecologists. *Amniocentesis and Chorionic Villus Sampling*. Green-top Guideline No. 8, June 2010.

45

You are performing a diagnostic laparoscopy on a 28-year-old woman with a body mass index (BMI) of 25 who has not had any previous surgery. You have introduced the Veress needle safely and started gas insufflations.

What intra-abdominal pressure should be achieved to safely insert the primary trocar?

a) 5–10 mmHg
b) 10–15 mmHg
c) 15–20 mmHg
d) 20–25 mmHg
e) 25–30 mmHg

Correct response: d

Explanation
A meta-analysis of the closed technique of entry showed that the risk of bowel damage was 0.4/1000 and the risk of major vessel injuries 0.2/1000. A pressure of 20–25 mmHg is recommended because the increased size of the 'gas bubble' has a splinting effect, which has been shown to be associated with a lower risk of major vessel injury. If a constant force of 3 kg is applied to the abdominal wall at the umbilicus to an abdominal cavity insufflated to a pressure of 10 mmHg, the depth under the 'indented' umbilicus is only 0.6 cm. With 25 mmHg, the depth is 5.6 cm (range 4–8 cm).

Royal College of Obstetricians & Gynaecologists. *Preventing Entry-related Gynaecological Laparoscopic Injuries*. Green-top Guideline No. 49, May 2008.

46

You have performed a hysteroscopy to investigate postmenopausal bleeding with a 5 mm hysteroscope, and while performing the curettage you suspect a uterine perforation.

What is the most appropriate management plan?

a) Administration of antibiotics and observation
b) Hysteroscopic repair
c) Laparoscopy
d) Laparotomy
e) Urgent postoperative imaging

Correct response: a

Explanation
Uterine perforation occurs in less than 1% of procedures but is more common in a pregnant uterus, during either a termination or an evacuation, especially if postpartum, and during operative hysteroscopy. The two principal dangers are bleeding and trauma. Lateral perforation is especially dangerous and can lead to significant bleeding, broad ligament haematoma, or rarely an arteriovenous malformation.

Shakir F, Diab Y. The perforated uterus. *The Obstetrician & Gynaecologist* 2013; **15**: 256–61.

47

A 35-year-old para 2 woman is referred to the gynaecology department with a history of worsening frequency, urgency and urge incontinence. There is no history of stress urinary incontinence, recurrent urinary tract infections, haematuria or prolapse symptoms. Urinalysis is normal.

Following a detailed history and examination, what would be the next most appropriate method of assessment?

a) Filling and voiding cystometry
b) Flexible cystoscopy
c) Renal tract ultrasound scan
d) Three-day bladder diary
e) Urine cytology

Correct response: d

Explanation
NICE advises that at the initial assessment the urinary incontinence (UI) symptoms should be categorized as stress UI, mixed UI or urgency UI/overactive bladder (OAB). Treatment should be started according to the predominant symptom. Bladder diaries should be part of the initial assessment of all women with UI or OAB. Urodynamic testing should only be performed after initiating conservative management.

National Institute for Health and Care Excellence (NICE). *Urinary Incontinence: the Management of Urinary Incontinence in Women.* NICE Clinical Guideline CG171, September 2013.

48

A 30-year-old woman is delivered at 27 weeks of gestation due to severe pre-eclampsia.

What is the risk of recurrence of severe pre-eclampsia in the subsequent pregnancy?

a) 20–25%
b) 30–35%
c) 40–45%
d) 50–55%
e) 60–65%

Correct response: d

Explanation
Recurrence following severe pre-eclampsia is common. Overall, the risk of recurrence is around 15% for women who had pre-eclampsia in one previous pregnancy and around 30% when two consecutive previous pregnancies were affected. It is much higher when pre-eclampsia is associated with a very preterm delivery. Counselling women who have had pre-eclampsia is an important part of a practising obstetrician's skills.

National Institute for Health and Care Excellence (NICE). *Hypertension in Pregnancy: the Management of Hypertensive Disorders during Pregnancy*. NICE Clinical Guideline CG107, August 2010.

49

A 45-year-old woman with symptomatic fibroids is considering uterine artery embolization (UAE). She has read that her symptoms might return after the procedure.

She should be informed that the risk of requiring further treatment for recurrent symptoms by five years is:

a) 5%
b) 10%
c) 15%
d) 20%
e) 25%

Correct response: b

Explanation
The risk is 25% by five years if < 40 years of age, but it reduces to 10% for those aged between 40 and 50 years.

Royal College of Obstetricians & Gynaecologists, Royal College of Radiologists. *Clinical Recommendations on the Use of Uterine Artery Embolisation (UAE) in the Management of Fibroids*, 3rd edition, 2013.

50

A primigravida was delivered by Neville Barnes forceps for a pathological cardiotocogram (CTG). Following delivery, a 3b perineal tear was diagnosed.

What is a 3b injury?

a) Both external and internal anal sphincters and anal epithelium torn
b) Both external and internal anal sphincters torn
c) Less than 50% of external anal sphincter thickness torn
d) More than 50% of external anal sphincter thickness torn
e) Perineal muscles torn

Correct response: d

Explanation
Accurate assessment of perineal tears is important, and adopting uniform definitions for perineal and anal sphincter injuries will allow more accurate audit and measurement of outcomes.

Royal College of Obstetricians & Gynaecologists. *The Management of Third- and Fourth-degree Perineal Tears*. Green-top Guideline No. 29, March 2007.

51

A 26-year-old woman has recently been diagnosed as being HIV positive. Her general practitioner notices that her first smear last year was negative, and contacts you for advice about the frequency of cervical smears for this woman.

How often should her cervical smears be undertaken?

a) Every 6 months
b) Every 6 months for 2 years and then routine recall
c) Annually
d) Every 3 years
e) Every 5 years

Correct response: c

Explanation

HIV alters the natural history of human papillomavirus (HPV) infection, with decreased regression rates and more rapid progression to high-grade and invasive lesions, which tend to be refractory to treatment. This requires more stringent intervention and monitoring.

NHS Cervical Screening Programme. *Colposcopy and Programme Management: Guidelines for the NHS Cervical Screening Programme*, 2nd edition. NHSCSP Publication No. 20, May 2010.

52

A 34-year-old woman is diagnosed to have vulval intraepithelial neoplasia grade 3 (VIN3) on a punch biopsy from a vulval lesion.

What is the recommended treatment for this condition?

a) Interferon therapy
b) Laser ablation of the lesion
c) Local surgical excision
d) Simple vulvectomy
e) Topical imiquimod cream

Correct response: c

Explanation

Local excision is adequate, with the same recurrence rates as more major surgery, and is considered the gold standard. It is possible to use non-surgical management, but careful follow-up is required. Laser ablation is not used in hair-bearing areas.

Royal College of Obstetricians & Gynaecologists. *The Management of Vulval Skin Disorders*. Green-top Guideline No. 58, February 2011.

53

A woman with a history of depression attends for pre-pregnancy counselling. She asks about antidepressant use in pregnancy.

Which is the antidepressant with the lowest known risk in pregnancy?

a) Amitriptyline
b) Fluoxetine
c) Nortriptyline
d) Paroxetine
e) Venlafaxine

Correct response: b

Explanation
It is important that clinicians discuss the use of these common drugs with women of childbearing years to ensure they are taking an appropriate drug. Tricyclic antidepressants (TCAs), such as amitriptyline, imipramine and nortriptyline, have lower known risks during pregnancy than other antidepressants. However, most TCAs have a higher fatal toxicity index than selective serotonin reuptake inhibitors (SSRIs). For this reason an SSRI is the drug of choice, and fluoxetine is the SSRI with the lowest known risk during pregnancy.

National Institute for Health and Care Excellence (NICE). *Antenatal and Postnatal Mental Health: Clinical Management and Service Guidance*. NICE Clinical Guideline CG45, February 2007 (recommendations 1.4.1.6 and 1.4.1.7).

54

A 56-year-old woman has been diagnosed with an overactive bladder (OAB).

What is the first line of treatment for this woman?

a) Bladder training for 6 weeks
b) Botulinum toxin injection into the bladder
c) OAB drug regime and bladder training
d) Percutaneous posterior tibial nerve stimulation
e) Transcutaneous sacral nerve stimulation

Correct response: a

Explanation
All women presenting with urinary incontinence should be offered supervised bladder training in the first instance with lifestyle advice. If this is not successful, an antimuscarinic can be added.

National Institute for Health and Care Excellence (NICE). *Urinary Incontinence: the Management of Urinary Incontinence in Women*. NICE Clinical Guideline CG171, September 2013 (recommendations 1.3 and 1.4).

55

A 37-year-old woman is seen in clinic after her third consecutive early pregnancy loss (miscarriage).

What is the most likely cause of recurrent miscarriage?

a) Antiphospholipid syndrome
b) Cervical factors
c) Genetic causes

d) Genital infections
e) Uterine anatomical abnormality

Correct response: a

Explanation
Antiphospholipid syndrome is the most common treatable cause of recurrent miscarriage. Antiphospholipid antibodies are present in 15% of women with recurrent miscarriage. The age-related risk of miscarriage at this age is 25%, rising to 93% when a woman reaches 45.

Royal College of Obstetricians & Gynaecologists. *The Investigation and Treatment of Couples with Recurrent First-trimester and Second-trimester Miscarriage*. Green-top Guideline No. 17, April 2011.

56

A community midwife asks for advice regarding a 20 weeks pregnant woman whose son has developed chickenpox a day before. The woman is not sure if she has had chickenpox herself. She is otherwise well.

What will be the most appropriate immediate management?

a) Ask her to come back if she develops any rash
b) Check varicella-zoster virus immunity and wait for result
c) Give varicella-zoster immunoglobulin as soon as possible
d) Reassure and do nothing, as she is completely asymptomatic
e) Treat with oral aciclovir for 7 days

Correct response: b

Explanation
The usual test turn-around time is 24–48 hours, and most of the women will be immune on testing. Varicella IgG is effective if given within 10 days of exposure. Pregnant women with chickenpox are at greater risk of morbidity and mortality, and pneumonia can occur in up to 10% of women with chickenpox. There is no risk to the fetus in the first trimester, but there is a small risk of varicella syndrome in babies if the infection is in the first 28 weeks of pregnancy. The most serious fetal risk is around term, and delivery should be delayed for five to seven days if possible to allow for the transfer of IgG antibodies.

Royal College of Obstetricians & Gynaecologists. *Chickenpox in Pregnancy*. Green-top Guideline No. 13, September 2007.

57

A 26-year-old primigravid woman attends the antenatal clinic at 12 weeks of gestation in view of a family history of a bleeding disorder. She too gives a history of a significant bleeding tendency, including spontaneous joint bleeds. A von Willebrand profile is performed and she is found to have unmeasurable von Willebrand factor (vWF) levels and severely low factor VIII (FVIII) levels.

What is the most likely diagnosis?

a) Haemophilia A
b) Haemophilia B
c) Type I von Willebrand's disease

d) Type 2a von Willebrand's disease
e) Type 3 von Willebrand's disease

Correct response: e

Explanation
It is only type 3 von Willebrand's disease (vWD) which gives you an unmeasurable vWF level, and consequently severely low FVIII levels. The other vWD types would not give such a severe bleeding tendency, and haemophilia typically affects males.

Pavord S. Inherited disorders of primary hemostasis. In Pavord S, Hunt B, eds., *The Obstetric Haematology Manual*. Cambridge: Cambridge University Press, 2010; pp. 176–85.

58

You are writing a guideline about prevention of venous thromboembolism (VTE) in pregnancy and you need to include information on background epidemiology.

What is the overall incidence of VTE in pregnancy and the puerperium?

a) 0.1–0.2/1000
b) 1–2/1000
c) 5–10/1000
d) 20–40/1000
e) 60–80/1000

Correct response: b

Explanation
The clinical diagnosis of VTE is difficult in pregnant women, but its prevalence is up to 10 times higher than in non-pregnant women of the same age. An obstetric unit with 5000 deliveries a year would expect to see 5–10 cases a year.

Royal College of Obstetricians & Gynaecologists. *Reducing the Risk of Thrombosis and Embolism during Pregnancy and the Puerperium*. Green-top Guideline No. 37a, November 2009.

59

A 34-year-old woman in her second pregnancy is seen in the antenatal clinic at 12 weeks. Three years ago she had a placental abruption resulting in a preterm delivery at 26 weeks. She has no other relevant history.

What is her risk of another abruption in this pregnancy?

a) 2–3%
b) 4–5%
c) 6–7%
d) 9–10%
e) 11–12%

Correct response: b

Explanation

History of abruption is the most predictive risk factor for abruption in a subsequent pregnancy. A 4.4% risk was reported in a large observational Norwegian study quoted in the RCOG guideline. It is important to be aware of this incidence so that a woman can be appropriately counselled.

Royal College of Obstetricians & Gynaecologists. *Antepartum Haemorrhage*. Green-top Guideline No. 63, November 2011.

60

A 19-year-old primigravida presents to the delivery suite in early labour. Her pregnancy has been low risk throughout. She is concerned about her delivery and would be very reluctant to consent to an operative vaginal delivery if she needed one.

Which of the following is most likely to increase her chances of achieving a spontaneous vaginal delivery?

a) Commencing pushing as soon as she is fully dilated
b) Continuous support in labour
c) Documenting progress on a partogram
d) Lying in the supine position during labour
e) Use of epidural for analgesia in labour

Correct response: b

Explanation

Continuous support in labour (especially by a non-member of staff) is known to decrease the need for a forceps/ventouse delivery, with a relative risk (RR) of 0.82. It helps to keep the woman upright or on her side during the second stage of labour. The use of epidural analgesia increases the risk of an operative vaginal delivery, with an odds ratio (OR) of 1.38.

Royal College of Obstetricians & Gynaecologists. *Operative Vaginal Delivery*. Green-top Guideline No. 26, January 2011.

61

A 28-year-old woman in her first pregnancy attends the antenatal clinic at eight weeks because of a strong family history of thromboembolism. Her general practitioner has performed a thrombophilia screen, which is reported as abnormal.

Which statement concerning the results of thrombophilia screening during pregnancy is correct?

a) Antithrombin levels are decreased
b) Factor V Leiden mutation cannot be diagnosed
c) Protein C levels are decreased
d) Protein S levels are decreased
e) Prothrombin gene mutation cannot be diagnosed

Correct response: d

Explanation

Antithrombin levels are unchanged during pregnancy; they only drop during labour. Factor V Leiden can be diagnosed during pregnancy by using a modified APC (activated protein C) resistance test. The pregnancy-induced changes in the thrombophilia screen take several weeks to return to the pre-pregnancy state. Protein C levels are unchanged during pregnancy; it is only protein S (both free and total) that drops.

Ramsay M. Normal haematological changes during pregnancy and the puerperium. In Pavord S, Hunt B, eds., *The Obstetric Haematology Manual*. Cambridge: Cambridge University Press, 2010; pp. 3–12.

62

A woman with a history of depression is referred for pre-conception counselling. She is concerned about her risk of postpartum psychosis.

From the following list, what is her risk of developing postpartum psychosis?

a) 2 per 1000
b) 3 per 1000
c) 4 per 1000
d) 5 per 1000
e) 6 per 1000

Correct response: a

Explanation

Postpartum depression occurs in 8–15% of women. About 0.1–2% of women develop postpartum psychosis. They have a 5% risk of suicide, and the infanticide rate is 5% if they are not treated. Suicide is a leading cause of maternal mortality. Women with bipolar disorder are at even higher risk from psychosis, with about a 1 in 4 risk of a severe recurrence.

Centre for Maternal and Child Enquiries (CMACE). Saving mothers' lives: reviewing maternal deaths to make motherhood safer: 2006–2008. The Eighth Report of the Confidential Enquiries into Maternal Deaths in the United Kingdom. *BJOG* 2011; **118** (Suppl. 1): 1–203 (Chapter 11: Deaths from psychiatric causes).
Di Florio A, Smith S, Jones I. Postpartum psychosis. *The Obstetrician & Gynaecologist* 2013; **15**: 145–50.
Edmonds DK. *Dewhurst's Textbook of Obstetrics and Gynaecology*, 8th edition. Chichester: Wiley, 2012.
Oates M. Psychiatric services for women following childbirth. *International Review of Psychiatry* 1996; **8**: 87–98.

63

The Confidential Enquiries into UK maternal deaths cover deaths directly and indirectly related to pregnancy.

The eighth report (2006–08) reported that the most common cause of indirect maternal death was:

a) Cardiac disease
b) Epilepsy
c) Hypertensive disease
d) Sepsis
e) Thromboembolism

Correct response: a

Explanation
The Confidential Enquiries report gives extensive information about maternal deaths in Britain. The top 10 recommendations provide advice on care standards. Causes of death change over time.

Centre for Maternal and Child Enquiries (CMACE). Saving mothers' lives: reviewing maternal deaths to make motherhood safer: 2006–2008. The Eighth Report of the Confidential Enquiries into Maternal Deaths in the United Kingdom. *BJOG* 2011; **118** (Suppl. 1): 1–203.

64
A 40-year-old woman underwent a LLETZ (large loop excision of the transformation zone) procedure in a hospital in England and the histology report showed incomplete excision of cervical intraepithelial neoplasia grade 3 (CIN3). Follow-up smear and human papillomavirus (HPV) testing at six months are negative.

What is the correct follow-up for this woman?

a) Annual smear for 10 years
b) Smear and HPV testing at 6 months
c) Smear and HPV testing at 12 months
d) Smear and HPV testing at 3 years
e) Smear and HPV testing at 5 years

Correct response: d

Explanation
The management guidelines reference the evidence used in their production, thus providing a useful resource in revision.

NHS Cervical Screening Programme. *Colposcopy and Programme Management: Guidelines for the NHS Cervical Screening Programme*, 2nd edition. NHSCSP Publication No. 20, May 2010.

65
You are called to obstetric theatre to see a woman who has a retained placenta. On examining her, you recognize that in addition to the retained placenta she has a partial uterine inversion. Your initial attempt to manually reduce the inversion is not successful.

What can the anaesthetist administer to assist you in reducing the inversion?

a) Carboprost 125 µg IV
b) Ergometrine 500 µg IV
c) Glycerine trinitrate 100 µg IV
d) Nifedipine 20 mg IV
e) Terbutaline 1 g IV

Correct response: c

Explanation
Glycerine trinitrate (GTN) causes uterine relaxation. Terbutaline can be used, but in a much lower dose than the dose described. In some cases a general anaesthetic is

necessary to reduce the inversion. Carboprost and ergometrine will make the uterus contract, and it will be even more difficult to replace.

Paterson-Brown S, Howell C, eds. *Managing Obstetric Emergencies and Trauma: the MOET Course Manual*. Cambridge: Cambridge University Press, 2014.

66

You see a 45-year-old nullipara in your gynaecology clinic who is a carrier for the *BRCA1* mutation. She wishes to discuss surgery to reduce her cancer risk.

What is the approximate average cumulative risk of her developing ovarian-type cancer by the age of 70?

a) 10%
b) 25%
c) 40%
d) 55%
e) 70%

Correct response: c

Explanation

BRCA mutations are autosomal dominant. In a family with both breast and ovarian cancers, 95% have *BRCA* mutations. The risk of ovarian cancer is lower with *BRCA2* at 11%. Many women will opt for ovarian surgery, in their 30s if they have *BRCA1* and in their 40s with *BRCA2*.

Antoniou A, Pharoah PD, Narod S, et al. Average risks of breast and ovarian cancer associated with *BRCA1* or *BRCA2* mutations detected in case series unselected for family history: a combined analysis of 22 studies. *American Journal of Human Genetics* 2003; **72**: 1117–30.

Devlin LA, Morrison PJ. Inherited gynaecological cancer syndromes. *The Obstetrician & Gynaecologist* 2008; **10**: 9–15.

67

You examine a 28-year-old primigravid woman in the antenatal ward at 36 weeks of gestation with polymorphic eruption of pregnancy, associated with generalized urticarial papules and increasingly severe pruritus. It has not responded to emollient creams, systemic antihistamines or topical steroids.

What further treatment is most likely to be effective?

a) Emollient creams
b) Intravenous immunoglobulins
c) Systemic aciclovir
d) Systemic prednisolone
e) Ultraviolet B phototherapy

Correct response: d

Explanation

Polymorphic eruption of pregnancy (PEP) is a distressing condition that occurs in between 1 in 160 and 1 in 300 pregnancies. It is usually seen in the third trimester and is associated with overdistension of the abdominal skin. It is self-limiting and usually resolves in four to six weeks. It is unusual to require oral steroids.

Vaughan Jones S, Ambros-Rudolph C, Nelson-Piercy C. Skin disease in pregnancy. *BMJ* 2014; **348**: g3489.

68

A primigravid woman is admitted for the medical management of early fetal demise at 15 weeks of gestation. She has received mifepristone 200 mg 48 hours prior to admission.

When prescribing her vaginal misoprostol, the total daily dosage should not exceed:

a) 400 µg
b) 800 µg
c) 1200 µg
d) 1600 µg
e) 2400 µg

Correct response: d

Explanation

Misoprostol is unlicensed in Britain but is widely used, supported by the World Health Organization (WHO) and by RCOG guidelines. The maximum total daily dose of misoprostol prescribed in the first trimester should be 2400 µg, reducing to 1600 µg from 13 to 17 weeks, and to 800 µg from 18 to 26 weeks in view of the increasing sensitivity of the uterus to prostaglandins.

Saraswat L, Ashok PW, Mathur M. Medical management of miscarriage. *The Obstetrician & Gynaecologist* 2014; **16**; 79–85.

69

A 40-year-old nulliparous woman is admitted with her fourth consecutive early pregnancy loss at 10 weeks of gestation.

A luteal-phase fall in which of these is associated with recurrent miscarriage?

a) Human chorionic gonadotrophin (hCG)
b) Insulin-like growth factor binding protein 1 (IGFBP1)
c) Oestradiol (E_2)
d) Prolactin (PRL)
e) Vitamin D

Correct response: a

Explanation

This is an association, probably related to the failing pregnancy. A meta-analysis published in 2013 showed a significant reduction in miscarriage rate in women treated with hCG. However, there was significant heterogeneity in the meta-analysis, and when the very early studies were removed and the heterogeneity reduced there was no significant difference. A large multicentre placebo-controlled trial was discontinued in the 1990s when an interim analysis showed no effect.

Morley L, Shillito J, Tang T. Preventing recurrent miscarriage of unknown aetiology. *The Obstetrician & Gynaecologist* 2013; **15**: 99–105.

70

A 32-year-old nulliparous woman presents to the gynaecology ward with an incomplete miscarriage. This is now her third consecutive early pregnancy loss.

Which investigation should routinely be carried out?

a) Cervical length estimation
b) Chlamydia test
c) Cytogenetic analysis of the products of conception
d) Parental chromosome tests
e) Thyroid function tests

Correct response: c

Explanation

Parental chromosome tests should only be performed when analysis of products of conception shows an abnormality.

Morley L, Shillito J, Tang T. Preventing recurrent miscarriage of unknown aetiology. *The Obstetrician & Gynaecologist* 2013; **15**: 99–105.

71

A 35-year-old woman attends your clinic for counselling regarding her risk of ovarian cancer. She has no family history of ovarian or breast cancer.

What is the lifetime risk of developing ovarian cancer in the general population?

a) < 1%
b) 1–2%
c) 3–4%
d) 5–6%
e) 7–8%

Correct response: b

Explanation

Approximately 1.4% of women will be diagnosed with ovarian cancer at some point during their lifetime, based on 2008–10 data.

National Cancer Institute. SEER stat fact sheet on ovarian cancer. http://seer.cancer.gov/statfacts/html/ovary.html (accessed 17 November 2014).

72

A 65-year-old woman is referred with an eight-month history of pain and itching in the vulval area. She is otherwise fit and well. You carry out a detailed clinical examination.

What appropriate investigation will you arrange to complement your clinical findings?

a) Blood tests and skin biopsy for all cases
b) Blood tests for autoimmune conditions if lichen planus is provisionally diagnosed
c) Blood tests for serum ferritin if vulval dermatitis is provisionally diagnosed
d) Blood tests for thyroid disorder and diabetes for all cases
e) Cervical smear if vulval intraepithelial neoplasia (VIN) is your clinical diagnosis

Correct response: c

Explanation
Evidence level 3: 20% of women with vulval dermatitis will have iron deficiency anaemia.

Royal College of Obstetricians & Gynaecologists. *The Management of Vulval Skin Disorders*. Green-top Guideline No. 58, February 2011.

73

During the labour ward handover, the coordinator informs you that there is a 35-year-old para 1 woman in labour with a face presentation. A junior doctor, who wants to do postgraduate training in obstetrics and gynaecology, is keen to learn more about this presentation.

What is the engaging diameter in a face presentation?

a) Bitemporal diameter
b) Occipito-frontal diameter
c) Submento-bregmatic diameter
d) Suboccipito-bregmatic diameter
e) Vertico-mental diameter

Correct response: c

Explanation
The chin being the denominator, the submento-bregmatic diameter is the presenting diameter in a face presentation, which is 9.5 cm.

Edmonds DK. *Dewhurst's Textbook of Obstetrics and Gynaecology*, 8th edition. Chichester: Wiley, 2012 (Chapter 26: Malpresentation, malposition, cephalopelvic disproportion and obstetric procedures).

74

A 26-year-old woman underwent surgical management of miscarriage and histopathology confirms normal trophoblast. Her last pregnancy, two years ago, was a molar pregnancy and she was followed up at the regional trophoblast screening centre.

What is the most appropriate follow-up, if any, in this pregnancy?

a) hCG level measurements in 4 weeks
b) hCG level measurements in 6 weeks
c) hCG level measurements monthly for 3 months
d) hCG level measurements monthly for 6 months
e) No follow-up

Correct response: b

Explanation
All women with a history of gestational trophoblastic disease should notify the screening centre at the end of any future pregnancy, whatever the outcome of the pregnancy. Human chorionic gonadotrophin (hCG) levels are measured six to eight weeks after the end of the pregnancy to exclude disease recurrence.

Royal College of Obstetricians & Gynaecologists. *The Management of Gestational Trophoblastic Disease*. Green-top Guideline No. 38, February 2010.

75

A 30-year-old primigravida presents in spontaneous labour at 41 weeks of gestation. On vaginal examination, the cervix is 8 cm dilated and the position of the vertex is left occipito-posterior.

What is the presenting diameter?

a) Bitemporal
b) Occipito-frontal
c) Submento-bregmatic
d) Suboccipito-bregmatic
e) Vertico-mental

Correct response: b

Explanation

Occipito-frontal diameter is the presenting diameter in occipto-posterior positions. Because the head is slightly extended this is 11.5 cm, which can lead to delay in the progress of labour.

Edmonds DK. *Dewhurst's Textbook of Obstetrics and Gynaecology*, 8th edition. Chichester: Wiley, 2012 (Chapter 26: Malpresentation, malposition, cephalopelvic disproportion and obstetric procedures).

76

You are attending a teaching session on labour management. You have been asked a series of questions regarding the mechanism by which the head is spontaneously born in a face presentation.

By what mechanism is the head delivered in a face presentation?

a) Extension
b) External rotation
c) Flexion
d) Internal rotation
e) Restitution

Correct response: c

Explanation

The mechanism of labour in a face presentation: descent, internal rotation, flexion, restitution and external rotation.

Edmonds DK. *Dewhurst's Textbook of Obstetrics and Gynaecology*, 8th edition. Chichester: Wiley, 2012 (Chapter 26: Malpresentation, malposition, cephalopelvic disproportion and obstetric procedures).

77

A 25-year-old woman requests emergency contraception following unprotected sexual intercourse on one occasion four days ago. She is currently taking a proton pump inhibitor for gastro-oesophageal reflux.

What emergency contraception would you recommend?

a) Copper intrauterine contraceptive device (IUCD)
b) Levonorgestrel (LNG)
c) LNG intrauterine system (Mirena coil)
d) Mifepristone
e) Ulipristal acetate (UPA)

Correct response: a

Explanation

UPA should not be used concomitantly with drugs that increase gastric pH. Mirena coil is not licensed for emergency contraception. LNG is recommended within 72 hours of unprotected intercourse. A copper IUCD can be used within five days of first unprotected intercourse in a cycle. Mifepristone is not licensed for emergency contraception in the UK.

Faculty of Sexual and Reproductive Healthcare. *Clinical Guidance: Emergency Contraception*, January 2012. http://www.fsrh.org/pdfs/CEUguidanceEmergencyContraception11.pdf (accessed 17 November 2014).

78

A 25-year-old woman is referred by the sexual health clinic due to an adnexal mass detected during copper coil insertion. She is symptom-free. A transvaginal scan shows a simple left ovarian cyst of 63 × 65 mm.

What would be your management plan?

a) MRI
b) Perform CA-125
c) Perform CA-125, LDH, AFP, hCG
d) Ultrasound after 6 months
e) Ultrasound after 12 months

Correct response: e

Explanation

A serum CA-125 assay does not need to be undertaken in all premenopausal women when an ultrasonographic diagnosis of a simple ovarian cyst has been made. Women with simple ovarian cysts of 50–70 mm in diameter should have yearly ultrasound follow-up.

Royal College of Obstetricians & Gynaecologists. *Management of Suspected Ovarian Masses in Premenopausal Women*. Green-top Guideline No. 62, November 2011.

79

You are asked to see a 40-year-old woman referred by the urologist because of an incidental finding of a simple right ovarian cyst measuring 43 × 47 mm on pelvic ultrasound. She has no gynaecological complaints.

What is your management plan?

a) CA-125 assay
b) CT scan
c) Gynaecological review in 3 months

d) No follow-up
e) Repeat ultrasound scan in 6 months

Correct response: d

Explanation
A serum CA-125 assay does not need to be undertaken in all premenopausal women when an ultrasonographic diagnosis of a simple ovarian cyst has been made. Women with small ovarian cysts (less than 50 mm diameter) generally do not require follow-up, as these are very likely to be physiological and almost always resolve within three menstrual cycles.

Royal College of Obstetricians & Gynaecologists. *Management of Suspected Ovarian Masses in Premenopausal Women*. Green-top Guideline No. 62, November 2011.

80

A 23-year-old woman in her first pregnancy with a history of systemic lupus erythematosus (SLE) attends for a detailed fetal anomaly ultrasound at 20 weeks of gestation. Autoantibody profile has detected Sjögren's syndrome A/B (anti-Ro/anti-La) antibodies.

What is the risk of the fetus developing congenital heart block?

a) 2–3%
b) 5–6%
c) 8–9%
d) 11–12%
e) 14–15%

Correct response: a

Explanation
It is important for obstetricians to be able to appropriately counsel patients regarding the risk to the fetus in the context of maternal SLE. Congenital heart block is associated with significant perinatal morbidity and mortality.

Cauldwell M, Nelson-Piercy C. Maternal and fetal complications of systemic lupus erythematosus. *The Obstetrician & Gynaecologist* 2012; **14**: 167–74.

81

A pregnant patient with thalassaemia books at the high-risk antenatal clinic at 10 weeks of gestation. She has a history of splenectomy. Her platelet count at booking is 650×10^9/L.

When considering her thrombotic risk, what treatment would you currently advise during pregnancy?

a) Low-dose aspirin 75 mg/day
b) Low-dose aspirin 75 mg/day and low-molecular-weight heparin (LMWH) therapeutic dose
c) Low-dose aspirin 75 mg/day and LMWH thromboprophylaxis
d) Use of TED anti-embolism compression stockings

e) Use of TED anti-embolism compression stockings and low-dose aspirin 75 mg/day

Correct response: c

Explanation
Patients with thalassaemia who have undergone splenectomy and have a platelet count > 600 × 10^9/L should be offered LMWH thromboprophylaxis as well as low-dose aspirin 75 mg/day. Women with thalassaemia major or intermedia have a prothrombotic tendency due to the presence of abnormal red cell fragments, especially if they have undergone splenectomy. These red cell fragments combined with a high platelet count significantly increase the risk of venous thromboembolism (VTE). This risk is highest in splenectomized women with thalassaemia intermedia who are not receiving transfusions, since a good transfusion regimen suppresses endogenous erythropoiesis.

Royal College of Obstetricians & Gynaecologists. *Management of Beta Thalassaemia in Pregnancy*. Green-top Guideline No. 66, March 2014.

82

A 35-year-old woman presents to the gynaecology clinic with left iliac fossa pain. Transvaginal ultrasound scan shows a 9 cm unilateral left ovarian mass, which is septated with echogenic foci. The right ovary cannot be identified separately and the uterus appears normal.

What are the most appropriate tumour markers to test in this case?

a) CA-125, AFP, hCG
b) CA-125, AFP, hCG, CEA
c) CA-125, AFP, hCG, LDH
d) CA-125, CEA, CA19-9
e) CA-125, CEA, LDH

Correct response: c

Explanation
Serum cancer antigen 125 (CA-125), alpha-fetoprotein (AFP), human chorionic gonadotrophin (hCG) and lactate dehydrogenase (LDH) should be measured in all premenopausal women under the age of 40 with a complex ovarian mass, as this could potentially represent a germ-cell tumour.

Royal College of Obstetricians & Gynaecologists. *Management of Suspected Ovarian Masses in Premenopausal Women*. Green-top Guideline No. 62, November 2011.

83

The United Kingdom Medical Eligibility Criteria (UKMEC) offers guidance to clinicians when considering the use of contraceptives. There are four categories, with Category 1 being generally suitable and Category 4 completely contraindicated.

When considering the combined oral contraceptive pill, which of the following factors would be considered as a Category 4 contraindication (i.e. completely contraindicated)?

a) Age 30 and smoking (more than 35/day)
b) Family history of breast cancer with a known *BRCA* gene mutation

c) History of deep venous thrombosis (DVT)
d) Hypertension 140/90 mmHg
e) Three weeks postnatal and breastfeeding

Correct response: e

Explanation
The decision to use any form of contraception is a decision a woman and her partner will make. If that includes the involvement of a clinician, they must weigh the advantages and disadvantages of the method chosen against the woman's medical and social history. A UK Category 1 indicates that there is no restriction for use. A UK Category 2 indicates that the method can generally be used, but more careful follow-up may be required. A contraceptive method with a UK Category 3 can be used, but this may require expert clinical judgement and/or referral to a specialist contraceptive provider, since use of the method is not usually recommended unless other methods are not available or not acceptable. A UK Category 4 indicates that use poses an unacceptable health risk.

Faculty of Sexual & Reproductive Healthcare. *UK Medical Eligibility Criteria for Contraceptive Use*, 2009. http://www.fsrh.org/pdfs/UKMEC2009.pdf (accessed 17 November 2014).

84

A 28-year-old para 1 woman with a history of polycystic ovary syndrome presents to the gynaecology emergency unit with a six-hour history of severe, intermittent left iliac fossa pain, nausea, vomiting and low-grade pyrexia. Transvaginal ultrasound scan suggests an enlarged oedematous left ovary with abnormal colour Doppler flow. Her white cell count is 16×10^9/L (normal 4–11), C-reactive protein 70 mg/L (normal < 10). She has been fluid resuscitated and has received intramuscular opioid analgesia.

What is the ideal management for this woman?

a) Admit to the inpatient ward for close observation
b) Diagnostic laparoscopy and de-torsion of left ovary
c) Diagnostic laparoscopy and left oopherectomy
d) Diagnostic laparoscopy and left partial oopherectomy
e) Explorative laparotomy

Correct response: b

Explanation
There is a high probability of ovarian torsion here. Surgery should be performed promptly to enable restoration of ovarian blood supply. Good outcome data exist to support conservative management with laparoscopy and de-torsion of ovary.

Damigos E, Johns J, Ross J. An update on the diagnosis and management of ovarian torsion. *The Obstetrician & Gynaecologist* 2012; **14**: 229–36.

85

A woman is readmitted 48 hours after a normal vaginal delivery. Symptoms and signs suggest profound septic shock.

What is the most appropriate first-line antibiotic regime to use?

a) Cefuroxime + metronidazole
b) Cefuroxime + metronidazole + gentamicin
c) Clindamycin + piperacillin/tazobactam
d) Co-amoxiclav + metronidazole
e) Co-amoxiclav + metronidazole + gentamicin

Correct response: c

Explanation
Clindamycin + piperacillin/tazobactam provides broad-spectrum cover in severe sepsis. It will cover most streptococci and staphylococci infections, and switch off exotoxin productions, with significantly decreased mortality. Cefuroxime should be avoided because of its association with *Clostridium difficile*.

Royal College of Obstetricians & Gynaecologists. *Bacterial Sepsis Following Pregnancy*. Green-top Guideline No. 64b, April 2012.

86

A 29-year-old woman is brought in to the emergency department by paramedics with a suspected pelvic fracture at 34 weeks of gestation after being hit by a car. She is hypotensive and tachycardic. She is being fluid resuscitated, and bloods including crossmatch have been sent.

What is the priority in the management of this woman?

a) Commence fetal monitoring in resuscitation
b) Immobilize the pelvis
c) Perform a full primary survey
d) Plan pelvic imaging and orthopaedic review
e) Plan transfer to labour ward for immediate delivery of baby

Correct response: c

Explanation
Pelvic fractures may bleed up to 3 litres, leading to circulatory collapse. There are likely to be other potentially life-threatening injuries. This patient needs a full primary survey to identify and treat these injuries, including rapid inspection to identify bleeding sites.

Paterson-Brown S, Howell C, eds. *Managing Obstetric Emergencies and Trauma: the MOET Course Manual*. Cambridge: Cambridge University Press, 2014.

87

A 47-year-old woman had a total abdominal hysterectomy for fibroids. Intraoperatively, deep retractor blades were used. She presents seven days postoperatively with weakness of hip flexion and adduction and knee extension. There is unilateral loss of knee jerk reflex and loss of sensation over the anteromedial thigh.

Which nerve is likely to have been injured intraoperatively?

a) Femoral nerve
b) Genitofemoral nerve
c) Ilioinguinal nerve

d) Lateral cutaneous nerve of the thigh
e) Obturator nerve

Correct response: a

Explanation
Nerve injury following gynaecological surgery is probably under-recognized, but faulty positioning of the patient, incisions, rectractor blades and specific surgery-related injuries lead to significant morbidity.

Kuponiyi O, Alleemudder DI, Latunde-Dada A, Eadarapalli P. Nerve injuries associated with gynaecological surgery. *The Obstetrician & Gynaecologist* 2014; **16**: 29–36.

88

A 38-week pregnant para 0 + 0 calls the maternity assessment department for advice. Her husband has been diagnosed with herpes zoster and she thinks she has not had chickenpox in the past.

What is the most appropriate management for this woman?

a) Check serology for varicella immunity
b) Give varicella-zoster immunoglobulin (VZIG)
c) Prescribe a course of aciclovir treatment
d) Reassure patient that she does not require treatment
e) Varicella vaccination

Correct response: a

Explanation
It is important to confirm immunity in the first instance. VZIG can be given up to 10 days after exposure, and usually serology will be reported within 24–48 hours.

Royal College of Obstetricians & Gynaecologists. *Chickenpox in Pregnancy*. Green-top Guideline No. 13, September 2007.

89

A 34-year-old woman is admitted for a diagnostic laparoscopy to investigate sub-fertility. She weighs 65 kg and is fit and healthy. The trainee performing the procedure is under direct supervision by the consultant.

At what angle to the skin should the primary trocar be inserted?

a) 15°
b) 30°
c) 45°
d) 60°
e) 90°

Correct response: e

Explanation
Entry at 90° ensures that the needle passes through the thinnest area of the abdominal wall where the peritoneum is firmly adherent to the underlying fascia.

Royal College of Obstetricians & Gynaecologists. *Preventing Entry-related Gynaecological Laparoscopic Injuries*. Green-top Guideline No. 49, May 2008.

90

A 28-year-old woman undergoes surgical termination of pregnancy at 13 weeks of gestation and sustains a uterine perforation.

Which one of the following is the instrument most commonly causing perforation?

a) Curette
b) Hegar dilator
c) Sponge-holding forceps
d) Suction cannula
e) Uterine sound

Correct response: d

Explanation

Suction cannula causes 51.3% of uterine perforations, Hegar dilator 24.4%, curette 16.2%.

Shakir F, Diab Y. The perforated uterus. *The Obstetrician & Gynaecologist* 2013; **15**: 256–61.

91

An 85-year-old woman has recently been diagnosed with vaginal carcinoma. The histology report confirmed squamous cell vaginal carcinoma and high prevalence of human papillomavirus (HPV).

Which type of HPV is responsible for the majority of vaginal carcinomas?

a) HPV-16
b) HPV-18
c) HPV-31
d) HPV-33
e) HPV-35

Correct response: a

Explanation

HPV-16 is responsible for the majority of HPV-related vaginal disease. HPV infection can render the whole lower genital tract vulnerable to neoplastic transformation.

Lippiatt J, Powell N, Tristram A. Non-cervical human papillomavirus-related disease. *The Obstetrician & Gynaecologist* 2013; **15**: 221–6.

92

A 28-year-old woman is in her third pregnancy. She is admitted for induction of labour for postdates. She is a known asthmatic and was admitted two weeks ago with exacerbation of asthma.

Which one of the following medications can be used safely for management of labour and postpartum?

a) Diclofenac
b) Ergometrine

c) Prostaglandin E_2
d) Prostaglandin $F_{2\alpha}$
e) Syntometrine

Correct response: c

Explanation
Syntometrine, ergometrine, prostaglandin F_{2a} (Haemabate), non-steroidal anti-inflammatory drugs and beta-blockers cause bronchospasm and should be used with caution.

Goldie MH, Brightling CE. Asthma in pregnancy. *The Obstetrician & Gynaecologist* 2013; **15**: 241–5.

93

Highly active antiretroviral therapy (HAART) in now routine in the management of HIV-positive women in pregnancy and is very effective in reducing mother-to-child transmission (MTCT) of HIV.

What is the incidence of transmission reduced to?

a) 0.1–0.5%
b) 1–2%
c) 3–5%
d) 6–8%
e) 9–11%

Correct response: b

Explanation
With the widespread implementation of routine antenatal screening for HIV-1, transmission of HIV-1 from mother to child is now a rare occurrence in the UK. The overall prevalence of HIV in pregnant women in the UK is highest in London, at 3.5/1000, and 1.6/1000 in the rest of England. The prevalence in sub-Saharan Africa has been stable over the last 10 years at 2–3%. The rate of HIV MTCT has reduced from 25.6% in 1993 to 1–2%. However, this is higher than it should be because of the small number of HIV-positive women who are undiagnosed at delivery. In treated women who have an undetectable viral load, the HIV MTCT is 0.1% (3/2000 in a study published in 2008).

British HIV Association guidelines for the management of HIV infection in pregnant women 2012. *HIV Medicine* 2012; **13** (Suppl. 2): 87–157. http://www.bhiva.org/documents/Guidelines/Pregnancy/2012/hiv1030_6.pdf (accessed 17 November 2014).

94

A 34-year-old nulliparous woman with asthma attends the antenatal clinic at 11 weeks of gestation. She is currently on regular salbutamol and steroid inhalers. She enquires regarding the effect of pregnancy on her asthma.

At what stage of pregnancy are exacerbations of asthma most common?

a) < 24 weeks
b) 24–36 weeks

c) > 36 weeks
d) During labour
e) In the postpartum period

Correct response: b

Explanation
Asthma is one of the many conditions in which a third will get worse, a third will get better and a third will see no change. Breathlessness in pregnancy is common, a physiological response to pregnancy, and may be interpreted as an exacerbation of asthma. Most exacerbations are triggered by a respiratory viral infection, but some are related to poor adherence to therapy.

Goldie MH, Brightling CE. Asthma in pregnancy. *The Obstetrician & Gynaecologist* 2013; **15**: 241–5.

95

A 28-year-old woman had a caesarean section for failure to progress. She visits her general practitioner four months postpartum with paraesthesia and sharp burning pains radiating from the incision site to the left labia and thigh.

Which nerve is most likely to have been involved?

a) Femoral nerve
b) Genitofemoral nerve
c) Iliohypogastric nerve
d) Lateral cutaneous nerve
e) Obturator nerve

Correct response: c

Explanation
Injuries to the iliohypogastric and ilioinguinal nerves are typically caused by suture entrapment at the lateral borders of the Pfannenstiel or low transverse incisions that extend beyond the lateral margin of the inferior rectus abdominis muscle.

Kuponiyi O, Alleemudder DI, Latunde-Dada A, Eadarapalli P. Nerve injuries associated with gynaecological surgery. *The Obstetrician & Gynaecologist* 2014; **16**: 29–36.

96

A 31-year-old nulliparous woman with HbSS is considering having a child with her partner, who has HbAS.

What is the probability that the child will have sickle cell disease?

a) 25%
b) 33%
c) 50%
d) 75%
e) 100%

Correct response: c

Explanation
In this case one partner has sickle cell disease (HbSS) while the other has sickle cell trait (HbAS), so 50% of their children will have sickle cell trait and 50% will have sickle cell disease.

Royal College of Obstetricians & Gynaecologists. *Management of Sickle Cell Disease in Pregnancy*. Green-top Guideline No. 61, July 2011.

97

A 29-year-old woman presents at 10 weeks of gestation with persistent vaginal bleeding and severe hyperemesis. On examination, the uterus is equivalent to 16 weeks in size. Ultrasound scan suggests a molar pregnancy. Uterine evacuation is performed under ultrasound guidance. She is registered to a UK screening centre to follow her gestational trophoblastic disease (GTD).

What is the optimum follow-up for GTD?

a) If human chorionic gonadotrophin (hCG) has reverted to normal within 28 days, follow-up will be for 6 months
b) If hCG has reverted to normal within 28 days, follow-up will be for 9 months
c) If hCG has reverted to normal within 28 days, follow-up will be for 12 months
d) If hCG has reverted to normal within 56 days, follow-up will be for 6 months
e) If hCG has reverted to normal within 56 days, follow-up will be for 9 months

Correct response: d

Explanation
Two large case series of just under 9000 cases have shown that, once hCG has normalized, the possibility of gestational trophoblastic neoplasia (GTN) developing is very low. GTN can occur after any GTD event, even when separated by a normal pregnancy.

Royal College of Obstetricians & Gynaecologists. *The Management of Gestational Trophoblastic Disease*. Green-top Guideline No. 38, February 2010.

98

A 41-year-old woman presents at 36 weeks of gestation in active labour. She has had a previous caesarean section and a subsequent precipitate vaginal delivery.

An ultrasound scan at 20 weeks showed a bilobed low-lying placenta. A repeat ultrasound scan at 32 weeks revealed a normally located placenta with polyhydramnios. Immediately after rupture of membranes, she started bleeding vaginally with associated cardiotocography (CTG) abnormalities.

What is the most likely diagnosis?

a) Abruptio placentae
b) Placenta accreta
c) Placenta percreta
d) Placenta praevia
e) Vasa praevia

Correct response: e

Explanation

Vasa praevia is a rare cause of vaginal bleeding but is associated with significant fetal morbidity and mortality. CTG changes in this situation would prompt a category 1 section.

Royal College of Obstetricians & Gynaecologists. *Placenta Praevia, Placenta Praevia Accreta and Vasa Praevia: Diagnosis and Management*. Green-top Guideline No. 27, January 2011.

99

A 28-year-old woman presents at 35 weeks in her second pregnancy feeling unwell, with backache, fever and rigors. She has a temperature of 39.5 °C. Her blood pressure is 60/40 mmHg, respiratory rate is 44 breaths/minute, pulse rate is 145 bpm. Speculum examination confirms foul-smelling vaginal discharge, and the serum lactate is > 4 mmol/L. She is not responding to the routine resuscitative measures.

What is the risk of maternal mortality?

a) 30%
b) 40%
c) 50%
d) 60%
e) 70%

Correct response: d

Explanation

Multi-organ dysfunction is associated with maternal mortality in the region of 20–40%, increasing to 60% if septic shock develops.

Royal College of Obstetricians & Gynaecologists. *Bacterial Sepsis in Pregnancy*. Green-top Guideline No. 64a, April 2012.

100

A diagnostic laparoscopy is being performed on a patient for suspected perforation of the uterus during suction evacuation of retained products of conception.

What is the most common site of uterine perforation?

a) Anterior
b) Fundus
c) Left lateral
d) Posterior
e) Right lateral

Correct response: a

Explanation

Site of uterine perforations in decreasing order: anterior wall (40%), cervical canal (36%), right lateral wall (21%), left lateral wall (17%), posterior wall (13%), fundus (13%).

Shakir F, Diab Y. The perforated uterus. *The Obstetrician & Gynaecologist* 2013; **15**: 256–61.

101

A 38-year-old woman has undergone a difficult laparoscopically assisted vaginal hysterectomy, with blood loss of 600 mL. Forty-eight hours after surgery, she complains of flank pain and has abdominal distension with generalized abdominal tenderness. She has oliguria and she is apyrexial. Bowel sounds are present but scanty. Investigations have revealed haemoglobin 10.8 g/L (normal 11.5–16.5), white cell count 8.3 × 10^9/L (normal 4–11) and creatinine 342 µmol/L (normal 27–88).

What is the most likely diagnosis?

a) Bowel injury
b) Ureteric injury
c) Urinary tract infection
d) Vault haematoma
e) Wound infection

Correct response: b

Explanation

Ureteric injury due to transection at surgery typically present 48 hours later (as opposed to thermal injury, which presents 10–14 days later). This case is suggestive of uroperitoneum; raised creatinine occurs due to reabsorption of urine from the peritoneum.

Minas V, Gul N, Aust T, Doyle M, Rowlands D. Urinary tract injuries in laparoscopic gynaecological surgery; prevention, recognition and management. *The Obstetrician & Gynaecologist* 2014; **16**: 19–28.

102

You are asked to review a woman eight hours after a vaginal delivery. She has an Obstetric Modified Early Warning Score of 6, which four hours previously was 0. She is tachycardic, tachypnoeic, hypotensive and pyrexial. She has abdominal tenderness and a sore throat.

What is the most likely causative organism?

a) *Clostridium septicum*
b) *Escherichia coli*
c) Group A *Streptococcus*
d) *Haemophilus influenzae*
e) *Staphylococcus aureus*

Correct response: c

Explanation

If symptoms develop within 12 hours of delivery, there is an associated sore throat, and rapid deterioration occurs, this is all suggestive of group A *Streptococcus* (GAS).

Royal College of Obstetricians & Gynaecologists. *Bacterial Sepsis Following Pregnancy*. Green-top Guideline No. 64b, April 2012.

103

You are investigating the effect of promoting immediate skin-to-skin contact at elective caesarean section and breastfeeding rates at six weeks postpartum. You have collected data over a period of six months on whether babies had immediate skin-to-skin contact and whether they were still being breastfed at six weeks.

What is the single most likely statistical test you would apply to the data to find a difference between the two groups?

a) ANOVA
b) Chi-squared
c) Odds ratio
d) Pearson's correlation
e) Student's *t*-test

Correct response: b

Explanation
A chi-squared test is used when testing to see if two factors are associated – in this situation, looking at the link between breast feeding and early skin-to-skin contact.

Petrie A, Sabin C. *Medical Statistics at a Glance*, 3rd edition. Chichester: Wiley, 2009.

104

A 30-year-old nulliparous woman has a cervical smear taken at her general practitioner's surgery as part of her routine screening recall. The result of the smear shows mild dyskaryosis. This is her first abnormal smear.

What is the appropriate management?

a) Offer prophylactic vaccination
b) Refer to a colposcopy clinic
c) Refer to a colposcopy clinic if she tests positive for high-risk HPV
d) Repeat the smear in 6 months
e) Repeat the smear in 24 months

Correct response: c

Explanation
Women who have low-grade dyskaryosis and who are positive for high-risk human papillomavirus (HR-HPV) must be referred for colposcopy. Women who are HR-HPV negative are returned to routine recall.

NHS Cervical Screening Programme. *Achievable Standards, Benchmarks for Reporting, and Criteria for Evaluating Cervical Cytopathology*, 3rd edition. NHSCSP Publication No. 1, January 2013.

105

A 34-year-old primigravida presents at 28 weeks of gestation with fever and flu-like symptoms with no gastrointestinal symptoms. She gives a history of recent travel to sub-Saharan Africa. Investigations confirm < 2% red blood cells parasitized with *Plasmodium falciparum*. She is clinically stable with no signs of severe infection. She has no drug allergies.

What is the most appropriate drug regime used for initial treatment?

a) Intravenous artesunate 2.4 mg/kg at 0, 12 and 24 hours followed by daily doses
b) Intravenous quinine 10 mg/kg TDS + IV clindamycin 450 mg TDS

c) Intravenous quinine 20 mg/kg loading dose followed by 10 mg/kg TDS + IV clindamycin 450 mgTDS
d) Oral quinine 600 mg followed by 300 mg 6–8 hours later
e) Oral quinine 600 mg TDS + oral clindamycin 450 mg TDS

Correct response: e

Explanation
Use quinine and clindamycin to treat uncomplicated *P. falciparum*.

Royal College of Obstetricians & Gynaecologists. *The Diagnosis and Treatment of Malaria in Pregnancy*. Green-top Guideline No. 54a, April 2010.
Royal College of Obstetricians & Gynaecologists. *The Prevention of Malaria in Pregnancy*. Green-top Guideline No. 54b, April 2010.

106

A 70-year-old woman had a sacrospinous fixation one week ago. She was readmitted complaining of severe right buttock and perineal pain, which is aggravated in the seating position.

What is the most likely nerve involvement?

a) Common peroneal nerve
b) Genitofemoral nerve
c) Ilioinguinal nerve
d) Obturator nerve
e) Pudendal nerve

Correct response: e

Explanation
The pudendal nerve (S2–S4) is susceptible to entrapment injuries during sacrospinous fixation as it runs behind the lateral aspect of the sacrospinous ligament.

Kuponiyi O, Alleemudder DI, Latunde-Dada A, Eadarapalli P. Nerve injuries associated with gynaecological surgery. *The Obstetrician & Gynaecologist* 2014; **16**: 29–36.

107

A 24-year-old primigravida presents at 24 weeks with increasing shortness of breath, orthopnoea and paroxysmal nocturnal dyspnoea. This was an unplanned pregnancy. She is known to have thalassaemia major, and her last blood transfusion was one week ago. Her current haemoglobin is 100 g/L.

Which is the most appropriate investigation for her?

a) Arterial blood gas (ABG)
b) Cardiac magnetic resonance imaging (MRI)
c) CT-guided pulmonary angiogram (CTPA)
d) Echocardiogram (ECHO)
e) Ventilation/perfusion scan (V/Q scan)

Correct response: b

Explanation
Cardiac failure is the primary cause of death in over 50% of all cases of thalassaemia major. This is due to cardiac dysfunction secondary to multiple transfusions. MRI will assess cardiac iron overload.

Royal College of Obstetricians & Gynaecologists. *Management of Beta Thalassaemia in Pregnancy*. Green-top Guideline No. 66, March 2014.

108

A 39-year-old woman has been referred with a history of three consecutive miscarriages. The first two miscarriages occurred before 10 weeks and the third was at 13 weeks of gestation. She has no significant medical history, and no uterine abnormalities were identified on a pelvic ultrasound scan.

What is the risk of miscarriage in the next pregnancy for this woman?

a) < 10%
b) 15–25%
c) 30–40%
d) 45–50%
e) 55–60%

Correct response: c

Explanation
The risk of miscarriage rises with age, doubling between 20 and 40. At the age of 36–39, the risk is 33%.

Royal College of Obstetricians & Gynaecologists. *The Investigation and Treatment of Couples with Recurrent First-trimester and Second-trimester Miscarriage*. Green-top Guideline No. 17, April 2011.

109

A 29-year-old nulliparous woman, suffering from cystic fibrosis, is contemplating pregnancy. Her sister-in-law recently had a baby with cystic fibrosis. Her partner is detected to be a carrier for cystic fibrosis.

What is the risk of the baby having cystic fibrosis?

a) 1/2
b) 1/4
c) 1/8
d) 1/25
e) 1/40

Correct response: a

Explanation
Cystic fibrosis is an autosomal recessive disorder. She will inevitably pass on the defective *CFTR* gene, and her partner has a 50% chance of passing on the defective copy.

Goddard J, Bourke SJ. Cystic fibrosis and pregnancy. *The Obstetrician & Gynaecologist* 2009; **11**: 19–24.

110

A 41-year-old primigravida is 14 weeks pregnant. She had in-vitro fertilization (IVF) and has a dichorionic and diamniotic twin pregnancy. She has chronic kidney disease and is attending the antenatal clinic for her first medical appointment.

Which one of her risk factors is the strongest predisposition for pre-eclampsia?

a) Age > 40 years
b) Chronic kidney disease
c) First pregnancy
d) IVF pregnancy
e) Multiple pregnancy

Correct response: b

Explanation

Fifty per cent of women with chronic kidney disease will develop hypertension by term, and 40% will develop significant proteinuria.

Edmonds DK. *Dewhurst's Textbook of Obstetrics and Gynaecology*, 8th edition. Chichester: Wiley, 2012.

National Institute for Health and Care Excellence (NICE). *Hypertension in Pregnancy: the Management of Hypertensive Disorders during Pregnancy*. NICE Clinical Guideline CG107, August 2010.

111

A 53-year-old woman had a total abdominal hysterectomy with bilateral salpingo-oophorectomy and omentectomy for a suspicious large ovarian cyst with raised CA-125. At laparotomy, it was noted that the tumour was limited to one ovary, but the capsule was breached. It was staged as Ic ovarian adenocarcinoma. The cytology for peritoneal washings was positive for adenocarcinoma cells.

What is the five-year survival?

a) 20%
b) 40%
c) 60%
d) 80%
e) 90%

Correct response: d

Explanation

FIGO staging for ovarian cancer:

I Growth limited to the ovaries
   Ia Tumour in one ovary; no ascites, capsule intact, no tumour on surface
   Ib As in Ia but tumour in both ovaries
   Ic Tumour either as in Ia or Ib, but ascites with cancer cells, or capsule ruptured or tumour on surface, or positive peritoneal washings
II Growth on one or both ovaries with peritoneal implants within the pelvis
   IIa Extension or metastases to uterus or fallopian tubes
   IIb Extension to other pelvic organs
   IIc Tumour either IIa or IIb, but with findings as in Ic

III Tumour in one or both ovaries with peritoneal implants outside the pelvis, or retroperitoneal node metastases
   IIIa Tumour grossly limited to the true pelvis; negative nodes, but microscopic implants on abdominal peritoneal surfaces
   IIIb As in IIIa, but abdominal implants are < 2 cm in diameter
   IIIc Abdominal implants > 2 cm, ± retroperitoneal lymph node metastases
IV Tumour involving one or both ovaries with distant metastases, e.g. malignant pleural fluid, parenchymal liver metastases

The overall five-year survival for stage I is 90%, but this is reduced to 80% in Ic because of the increased risk of recurrence due to breach of the ovarian capsule.

Edmonds DK. *Dewhurst's Textbook of Obstetrics and Gynaecology*, 8th edition. Chichester: Wiley, 2012.

112

A 27-year-old woman attends antenatal clinic at 29 weeks of gestation and is found to have a blood pressure of 148/99 mmHg. Testing her urine shows ++ of proteinuria. She is asymptomatic.

What is the most appropriate initial management?

a) Admit to hospital for observation
b) Arrange for the community midwife to visit the patient at home in 24 hours
c) Commence methyldopa 250 mg three times a day and follow up on day assessment unit in 48 hours
d) Commence treatment with labetalol 200 mg three times a day and follow up on day assessment unit in 48 hours
e) Refer to day assessment unit for blood pressure profile and further assessment

Correct response: a

Explanation
In pre-eclampsia with mild hypertension (140–149/90–99 mmHg) the National Institute for Health and Care Excellence (NICE) recommends admission to hospital but not treatment, daily bloods or proteinuria quantification.

National Institute for Health and Care Excellence (NICE). *Hypertension in Pregnancy: the Management of Hypertensive Disorders during Pregnancy*. NICE Clinical Guideline CG107, August 2010.

113

A 30-year-old woman had a 3c perineal tear at her first vaginal delivery. She attends the postnatal perineal trauma clinic at six weeks. She is concerned about her persistent symptom of faecal urgency.

What percentage of women are asymptomatic at 12 months after sustaining a third-degree tear?

a) 1–20%
b) 21–40%
c) 41–60%
d) 61–80%
e) 81–100%

Correct response: d

Explanation

Outcome following primary repair of third- and fourth-degree perineal tears is good.

Royal College of Obstetricians & Gynaecologists. *The Management of Third- and Fourth-degree Perineal Tears*. Green-top Guideline No. 29, March 2007.

114

A 49-year-old woman attends the urogynaecology clinic with symptoms of frequency, urgency and nocturia. She has already had bladder training. Her urinalysis is negative for infection.

What of the following is the next level of management?

a) Mirabegron
b) Pelvic floor exercises
c) Sacral nerve stimulation
d) Trospium
e) Urodynamic investigations

Correct response: d

Explanation

After bladder training, oxybutynin, trospium or darifenacin is considered. Mirabegron is a beta-2 agonist that is considered after failure of antimuscarinics. Sacral nerve stimulation is the final option for treatment, owing to its cost and invasive nature.

National Institute for Health and Care Excellence (NICE). *Urinary Incontinence: the Management of Urinary Incontinence in Women*. NICE Clinical Guideline CG171, September 2013.

115

A low-risk primigravida is admitted in spontaneous labour at term with intact membranes. She is contracting strongly, four in 10 minutes. The cervix is effaced and 5 cm dilated, cephalic presentation, occipito-anterior position with no caput or moulding and 1 cm above the ischial spines. Four hours later, she is 6 cm dilated. All other findings are unchanged. Intermittent auscultation is normal.

According to National Institute for Health and Care Excellence (NICE) guidance, what is the diagnosis and recommended management?

a) Adequate progress in the first stage, vaginal examination in 4 hours
b) Confirmed delay in the first stage, amniotomy and vaginal examination in 2 hours
c) Confirmed delay in the first stage, amniotomy and vaginal examination in 4 hours
d) Suspected delay in the first stage, amniotomy and vaginal examination in 2 hours
e) Suspected delay in the first stage, amniotomy and vaginal examination in 4 hours

Correct response: d

Explanation

Suspected delay is < 2 cm progress in four hours; amniotomy should be offered. If < 1 cm progress on vaginal examination in two hours, this is confirmed delay in the first stage.

National Institute for Health and Care Excellence (NICE). *Intrapartum Care: Care of Healthy Women and Their Babies During Childbirth*. NICE Clinical Guideline CG55, September 2007.

116

A 90-year-old woman with multiple comorbidities has a vault prolapse that cannot be managed with a shelf pessary. She is struggling with the repeated hospital visits and examinations and requests definitive treatment.

Which surgical procedure is best suited to this woman?

a) Abdominal sacrocolpopexy
b) Burch colposuspension
c) Colpocleisis
d) Posterior intravaginal slingplasty
e) Vaginal uterosacral ligament suspension

Correct response: c

Explanation

Colpocleisis is ideal for frail elderly ladies who do not wish to retain their sexual function. It has low complication rates and high success rates.

Royal College of Obstetricians & Gynaecologists. *The Management of Post Hysterectomy Vaginal Vault Prolapse*. Green-top Guideline No. 46, October 2007.

117

A 45-year-old woman is due to have a transobturator tape procedure for stress urinary incontinence. You counsel her about the risks of the procedure, including the risk of obturator nerve injury.

What motor findings would be consistent with obturator nerve injury?

a) Weakness of hip extension
b) Weakness of hip external rotation
c) Weakness of hip flexion
d) Weakness of thigh abduction
e) Weakness of thigh adduction

Correct response: e

Explanation

The obturator nerve arises from L2–L4, provides sensation to the upper medial thigh and is responsible for thigh adduction. Damage usually presents with minor problems on walking.

Kuponiyi O, Alleemudder DI, Latunde-Dada A, Eadarapalli P. Nerve injuries associated with gynaecological surgery. *The Obstetrician & Gynaecologist* 2014; 16: 29–36.

118

A 30-year-old primiparous woman attends pre-conception counselling prior to undergoing in-vitro fertilization (IVF) treatment, because of a strong family history of venous thromboembolism in several first-degree relatives. She has a body mass index (BMI) of 34 and has no previous major medical problems.

Which blood test would be most helpful in determining her management?

a) Anti-Xa levels
b) Anticardiolipin antibodies
c) Lupus anticoagulant
d) Methyltetrahydrofolate reductase genotype
e) Thrombophilia screen

Correct response: e

Explanation

The key point in this question is to recognize that the family history raises the possibility of a heritable thrombophilia, which requires a thrombophilia screen to detect.

Royal College of Obstetricians & Gynaecologists. *Reducing the Risk of Thrombosis and Embolism during Pregnancy and the Puerperium*. Green-top Guideline No. 37a, November 2009.

119

A 29-year-old primigravida presents with an intrauterine fetal death at 26 weeks. She has been feeling unwell for a few days. She has intact membranes but the liquor is noted to be green at delivery.

What is the most likely cause of this fetal loss?

a) Cytomegalovirus
b) Group A *Streptococcus*
c) Group B *Streptococcus*
d) *Listeria monocytogenes*
e) Parvovirus B19

Correct response: d

Explanation

Listeriosis is an uncommon disease in the healthy immunocompetent population but is 17 times more common in pregnancy. Although the same serotypes can affect animals and humans, most human infection is from contaminated food. Infection is transplacental or may be an ascending infection from the vagina. Preterm fetal loss with green liquor is a classic finding in *Listeria* infection.

Royal College of Obstetricians & Gynaecologists. *Late Intrauterine Fetal Death and Stillbirth*. Green-top Guideline No. 55, October 2010.

120

A 35-year-old woman with known myasthenia gravis attends for pre-conception counselling.

Which of the following drugs should be avoided in pregnancy?

a) Azathioprine
b) Ciclosporin

c) Mycophenolate mofetil
d) Prednisolone
e) Pyridostigmine

Correct response: c

Explanation
Mycophenolate mofetil is the most teratogenic, and is advised to be discontinued prior to pregnancy. There is an increased risk of first-trimester pregnancy loss, and of confirmed human teratogenic effects including cleft lip and/or palate, microtia, micrognathia and hypertelorism.

UK Teratology Information Service. http://www.uktis.org (accessed 17 November 2014).

121

A 27-year-old woman presents in labour having had no antenatal care in the UK. She informs the midwife that she is HIV positive. She has had no antiretroviral treatment in her pregnancy.

What is the risk of vertical transmission with no intervention in this case?

a) 5–10%
b) 15–20%
c) 25–30%
d) 35–40%
e) 45–50%

Correct response: c

Explanation
Untreated HIV: 25–30% transmission to fetus in utero. Treated HIV: approximately 8% transmission to fetus in utero. Untreated HIV: 50–60% transmission to baby during breastfeeding.

British HIV Association guidelines for the management of HIV infection in pregnant women 2012. *HIV Medicine* 2012; **13** (Suppl. 2): 87–157. http://www.bhiva.org/documents/Guidelines/Pregnancy/2012/hiv1030_6.pdf (accessed 17 November 2014).

122

A 49-year-old woman attends for outpatient hysteroscopy to investigate abnormal vaginal bleeding.

What intervention is routinely recommended to reduce procedure-related pain?

a) Dihydrocodeine pre-procedure
b) Instillation of local anaesthetic gel into the cervical canal pre-procedure
c) Misoprostol pre-procedure
d) Non-steroidal anti-inflammatory drugs pre-procedure
e) Paracervical block with local anaesthetic pre-procedure

Correct response: d

Explanation
Instillation of local anaesthetic into the cervical canal does not reduce pain during diagnostic outpatient hysteroscopy but may reduce the incidence of vasovagal reactions.

Royal College of Obstetricians & Gynaecologists. *Best Practice in Outpatient Hysteroscopy*. Green-top Guideline No. 59, March 2011.

123

A 58-year-old postmenopausal woman presents with pelvic pain and a persistent 6 cm simple unilocular left ovarian cyst on pelvic ultrasound. Her CA-125 is 25 IU/mL. She opts for surgical management.

What is the most appropriate surgical management?

a) Aspiration of the cyst
b) Bilateral oophorectomy
c) Left oophorectomy
d) Left ovarian cystectomy
e) Total hysterectomy, bilateral salpingo-oophorectomy and omentectomy

Correct response: b

Explanation
Although unilateral oophorectomy may be performed if that is the patient's wish, it is considered safer to remove both ovaries if possible. The ovaries should be removed intact into a bag, avoiding rupture.

Royal College of Obstetricians & Gynaecologists. *Ovarian Cysts in Postmenopausal Women*. Green-top Guideline No. 34, October 2003, reviewed 2010.

124

A 46-year-old woman had a total abdominal hysterectomy for heavy menstrual bleeding due to fibroids. She had defaulted many years ago from the routine recall for cervical smears but this was not picked up before the operation. Histology showed no cervical intraepithelial neoplasia (CIN) in the hysterectomy specimen.

What is the most appropriate follow-up?

a) No further cytology required
b) Vaginal vault cytology immediately
c) Vaginal vault cytology at 6 weeks
d) Vaginal vault cytology at 6 months
e) Vaginal vault cytology at 6 months and 18 months

Correct response: d

Explanation
Although the specimen shows no abnormality, the woman should have a vault smear six months following surgery. The responsibility for informing the woman and her general practitioner rests with the gynaecologist performing the surgery.

NHS Cervical Screening Programme. *Colposcopy and Programme Management: Guidelines for the NHS Cervical Screening Programme*, 2nd edition. NHSCSP Publication No. 20, May 2010.

125

A 20-year-old primigravida has an incidental finding of cervical length of 20 mm at her routine 20-week anomaly scan. She is asymptomatic and has no significant past medical or surgical history.

What is the most appropriate management?

a) Abdominal cerclage
b) Cervical cerclage
c) Counsel the woman that no further action is required
d) Progesterone pessaries
e) Serial ultrasound scan to assess cervical length

Correct response: c

Explanation

If there is no previous history of preterm labour or second-trimester loss, the incidence of preterm labour is not reduced by inserting a cerclage.

Royal College of Obstetricians & Gynaecologists. *Cervical Cerclage*. Green-top Guideline No. 60, May 2011.

126

A primigravid woman has been having serial ultrasound scans for a small-for-gestational-age fetus. The fetal biometry is below the 10th centile, with normal liquor volumes and umbilical artery Doppler. She reports good fetal movements. She is currently 37 weeks pregnant and has declined induction of labour.

After appropriate counselling regarding risks to her baby, what is the most appropriate management for this woman?

a) Admit her for observation
b) Cardiotocography weekly
c) Cardiotocography twice weekly
d) Umbilical artery Doppler and liquor volume weekly
e) Umbilical artery Doppler and liquor volume twice weekly

Correct response: d

Explanation

The recommendation would be to induce at 37 weeks, but if she refuses induction, umbilical artery Doppler should be the primary surveillance tool. It has been shown to reduce perinatal morbidity and mortality. At an earlier gestation, fortnightly review would be appropriate.

Royal College of Obstetricians & Gynaecologists. *The Investigation and Management of the Small-for-Gestational-Age Fetus*, 2nd edition. Green-top Guideline No. 31, February 2013.

127

A 36-year-old woman has attended for pre-conception counselling. She has a history of systemic lupus erythematosus for the last 15 years. Her first child, now two years old, had a pacemaker fitted for congenital heart block.

What is the risk of heart block in subsequent pregnancy?

a) 5%
b) 15%
c) 25%
d) 35%
e) 50%

Correct response: b

Explanation

The risk of recurrence of congenital heart block due autoimmune causes is around 15%.

Nelson-Piercy C. Autoimmune conditions. In Luesley DM, Baker PN, eds., *Obstetrics and Gynaecology: an Evidence-based Text for MRCOG*, 2nd edition. London: E. Arnold, 2010, pp. 92–7.

128

A 25-year-old woman attends the postnatal clinic. She delivered her son eight weeks ago at 27 weeks of gestation following an eclamptic seizure. She is keen to have further children.

What is her risk of pre-eclampsia in her next pregnancy?

a) 5%
b) 10%
c) 25%
d) 50%
e) 75%

Correct response: d

Explanation

National Institute for Health and Care Excellence (NICE) guidelines state that there is a risk of pre-eclampsia in subsequent pregnancies of 1 in 4 if the severe pre-eclampsia/HELLP syndrome/eclampsia leading to birth occurred at less than 34 weeks, and 1 in 2 if it occurred at less than 28 weeks.

National Institute for Health and Care Excellence (NICE). *Hypertension in Pregnancy: the Management of Hypertensive Disorders during Pregnancy*. NICE Clinical Guideline CG107, August 2010.

129

A 25-year-old pregnant woman with sickle cell disease and a history of previous transfusion is blood group B negative. She has anti-D antibodies. She requires a non-emergency blood transfusion.

Which blood would be suitable for transfusion?

a) B negative, CMV negative, Kell negative
b) B negative, CMV negative, Kell positive
c) B negative, CMV positive, Kell positive
d) B positive, CMV negative, Kell negative
e) B positive, CMV positive, Kell positive

Correct response: a

Explanation
Pregnant women should always receive cytomegalovirus (CMV)-seronegative and Kell-negative blood. Kell is associated with a high risk of alloimmunization, and blood should be seronegative for CMV unless CMV status is known.

Royal College of Obstetricians & Gynaecologists. *Blood Transfusions in Obstetrics.* Green-top Guideline No. 47, December 2007.
Royal College of Obstetricians & Gynaecologists. *The Management of Women with Red Cell Antibodies during Pregnancy.* Green-top Guideline No. 65, May 2014.

130

A 35-year-old woman is admitted to hospital at 34 weeks of gestation with a worsening of her asthma.

Approximately what proportion of women experience a deterioration of their asthma in pregnancy?

a) 10%
b) 30%
c) 50%
d) 60%
e) 75%

Correct response: b

Explanation
Between 30% and 35% of women will experience a deterioration of their asthma in pregnancy, and 23% will see an improvement. If asthma is well controlled, there is little or no increase in maternal or fetal complication. If poorly controlled, there is an association with hyperemesis, hypertension, pre-eclampsia, vaginal bleeding, complicated labour, fetal growth restriction, preterm delivery, increased perinatal morbidity and mortality, and increased caesarean section rate.

British Thoracic Society, Scottish Intercollegiate Guidelines Network. *British Guideline on the Management of Asthma.* SIGN 141, October 2014. http://sign.ac.uk/guidelines/fulltext/141 (accessed 17 November 2014).

131

A 27-year-old woman with epilepsy attends antenatal clinic in the third trimester of pregnancy. She is well controlled on lamotrigine.

In women with treated epilepsy, what is the risk of having a tonic–clonic seizure in the peripartum period?

a) 1–5%
b) 10–15%
c) 20–25%
d) 30–35%
e) 40–45%

Correct response: a

Explanation

The guidelines state that the risk of tonic–clonic seizures during labour and in the 24 hours after birth is low (1–4%).

National Institute for Health and Care Excellence (NICE). *The Epilepsies: the Diagnosis and Management of the Epilepsies in Adults and Children in Primary and Secondary Care*. NICE Clinical Guideline CG137, January 2012 (section 1.15: Women and girls with epilepsy).

132

A 24-year-old woman in her first pregnancy has been diagnosed with hydrops fetalis on her anomaly scan at 20 weeks of gestation. Maternal serology is negative for immune causes.

What is the risk of fetal mortality without intervention in non-immune hydrops fetalis?

a) 20%
b) 40%
c) 60%
d) 80%
e) 100%

Correct response: d

Explanation

Non-immune hydrops fetalis carries a very poor prognosis, especially when detected early in pregnancy. The incidence of fetal death is 75–90%. There are many causes, including infections (e.g. parvovirus B19, cytomegalovirus, syphilis), aneuploidies, fetal cardiac anomalies, neurological disorders and gastrointestinal disorders of the fetus, although in 30–50% of fetuses a definite diagnosis is not made.

To M, Kidd M, Maxwell D. Prenatal diagnosis and management of fetal infections. *The Obstetrician & Gynaecologist* 2009; **11**: 108–16.

133

You are working as a year 4 specialist trainee. You have a meeting with your educational supervisor in which your achievements and challenges over the last four months are discussed. You jointly plan specific objectives to achieve over the next four months, including a clinical audit and attending a postgraduate course.

How would you best describe this encounter?

a) Appraisal
b) Mini clinical evaluation exercise
c) Revalidation

d) Summative assessment
e) Team observation

Correct response: a

Explanation
Appraisal reviews personal and educational development and is not measured against any set criteria, nor does it contribute to a formal summative assessment. Appraisal is jointly developed by the trainee and trainer and should lead to a personal development plan. Summative assessment occurs when a pass/fail decision is made, depending on results.

Shehmar M, Khan KS. A guide to the ATSM in Medical Education. Article 2: assessment, feedback and evaluation. *The Obstetrician & Gynaecologist* 2010; **12**: 119–25.

134

A 22-year-old woman is on the postnatal ward having had a normal delivery. The midwife notices that the baby has sticky eyes on the morning after delivery.

What is the most common causative organism of infective neonatal conjunctivitis?

a) *Chlamydia trachomatis*
b) *Haemophilus influenzae*
c) *Neisseria gonorrhoeae*
d) *Staphylococcus aureus*
e) *Streptococcus pneumoniae*

Correct response: a

Explanation
C. trachomatis is the commonest single cause of neonatal conjunctivitis in industrially developed countries (up to 40% of cases). An infant born to a mother with *Chlamydia* has a 30–40% chance of developing conjunctivitis. Non-sexually transmitted bacteria such as *Staphylococcus*, *Streptococcus* and *Haemophilus* species, and other Gram-negative bacteria, make up most of the remaining cases (30–50%). *N. gonorrhoeae* causes less than 1% of cases of neonatal conjunctivitis.

National Institute for Health and Care Excellence (NICE). Conjunctivitis – infective. Scenario: neonatal conjunctivitis. NICE Clinical Knowledge Summaries, August 2012. http://cks.nice.org.uk/conjunctivitis-infective#!scenario:2 (accessed 17 November 2014).
Zar HJ. Neonatal chlamydial infections. *Pediatric Drugs* 2005; **7**: 103–10.

135

Following instrumental vaginal delivery, vaginal and rectal examination shows a perineal tear involving less than 50% of the external anal sphincter. The internal anal sphincter and rectal mucosa are intact.

What is the classification of this perineal injury?

a) Second degree
b) Third degree: 3a
c) Third degree: 3b

d) Third degree: 3c
e) Fourth degree

Correct response: b

Explanation
Third-degree injury to perineum involving the anal sphincter complex:

3a Less than 50% of external anal sphincter thickness torn
3b More than 50% of external anal sphincter thickness torn
3c Both external and internal anal sphincter torn

Royal College of Obstetricians & Gynaecologists. *The Management of Third- and Fourth-degree Perineal Tears*. Green-top Guideline No. 29, March 2007.

136

You have performed a diagnostic hysteroscopy which was complicated by a uterine perforation. You complete a clinical adverse incident report and later review the case to identify any gaps in your knowledge or skills. You record and discuss your thoughts with your educational supervisor.

How would you best describe this learning exercise?

a) Appraisal
b) Mini clinical evaluation exercise
c) Reflective practice
d) Risk assessment
e) Root cause analysis

Correct response: c

Explanation
Reflective practice is a structured way of thinking during and after events in our clinical practice in order to enhance safety and highlight needs in our learning. Reflective practice is an effective process to analyse and identify continuing professional development needs.

Royal College of Obstetricians & Gynaecologists. StratOG eLearning. https://stratog.rcog.org.uk (accessed 17 November 2014).

137

You are performing a diagnostic laparoscopy. You have placed the primary trocar following carbon dioxide insufflation with a Veress needle.

What is the recommended range of intra-abdominal pressure for insertion of the secondary trocar under direct vision?

a) 5–10 mmHg
b) 10–15 mmHg
c) 15–20 mmHg
d) 20–25 mmHg
e) 25–30 mmHg

Correct response: d

Explanation
A pressure of 20–25 mmHg results in increased splinting and allows the trocar to be more easily inserted through the layers of the abdominal wall. The increased size of the 'gas bubble' and this splinting effect has been shown to be associated with a lower risk of major vessel injury.

Royal College of Obstetricians & Gynaecologists. *Preventing Entry-related Gynaecological Laparoscopic Injuries*. Green-top Guideline No. 49, May 2008.

138

A 23-year-old woman undergoes a surgical evacuation for a suspected molar pregnancy. Histology has confirmed a partial mole.

What is the most common chromosomal composition of a partial mole?

a) 1 paternal and 1 maternal gametes
b) 1 paternal and 2 maternal gametes
c) 2 paternal and 1 maternal gametes
d) 2 paternal and no maternal gametes
e) 3 paternal and 1 maternal gametes

Correct response: c

Explanation
Partial moles are usually (90%) triploid in origin, with two sets of paternal haploid chromosomes and one set of maternal haploid chromosomes. Partial moles occur, in almost all cases, following dispermic fertilization of an ovum. Ten per cent of partial moles represent tetraploid or mosaic conceptions.

Royal College of Obstetricians & Gynaecologists. *The Management of Gestational Trophoblastic Disease*. Green-top Guideline No. 38, February 2010.
Savage P. Molar pregnancy. *The Obstetrician & Gynaecologist* 2008; **10**: 3–8.

139

A 60-year-old postmenopausal woman presents to the gynaecology clinic with a history of gradual onset of vulval itching and burning. She has suffered from urinary incontinence for two years. Examination reveals vulval erythema and scaling.

What is the most likely diagnosis?

a) Irritant dermatitis
b) Lichen planus
c) Lichen sclerosus
d) Paget's disease
e) Squamous cell carcinoma

Correct response: a

Explanation
Although lichen sclerosus is a common cause of vulval itching, it does not cause erythema and scaling. Common irritants include panty liners, detergents, lubricants and urinary incontinence.

Kingston A. The postmenopausal vulva. *The Obstetrician & Gynaecologist* 2009; **11**: 253–9.

140

A 31-year-old woman is diagnosed with a missed miscarriage at 11 weeks in her first pregnancy. Her body mass index (BMI) is 26 and she has no medical history. She wants to know the reason for the miscarriage.

What is the most common cause of first-trimester miscarriage?

a) Fetal aneuploidy
b) Infection
c) Smoking
d) Thrombophilia
e) Uterine anomaly

Correct response: a

Explanation
Most first-trimester miscarriages are related to fetal aneuploidy, which the woman cannot affect, but advice on smoking, weight and any other factor that she can affect should be discussed.

National Institute for Health and Care Excellence (NICE). *Ectopic Pregnancy and Miscarriage: Diagnosis and Initial Management in Early Pregnancy of Ectopic Pregnancy and Miscarriage*. NICE Clinical Guideline CG154, December 2012.

141

A 39-year-old woman has a normal delivery of her third baby. She requests long-term contraception. She has previously used a copper intrauterine device but has a history of menorrhagia. You counsel her about a levonorgestrel-releasing intrauterine system (Mirena coil).

What is the recommended time interval for insertion of the levonorgestrel-releasing system following delivery?

a) 7 days
b) 14 days
c) 21 days
d) 28 days
e) 42 days

Correct response: d

Explanation
There is an increased risk of perforation following insertion prior to 28 days. If she is not breastfeeding, she is likely to ovulate before six weeks.

Faculty of Sexual & Reproductive Healthcare. *Postnatal Sexual and Reproductive Health*, September 2009. http://www.fsrh.org/pdfs/CEUguidancepostnatal09.pdf (accessed 17 November 2014).

142

A 26-year-old woman has pelvic girdle pain and has been booked for induction of labour at 39 weeks. She is diagnosed with primary varicella-zoster virus at 38 + 6 weeks of gestation.

What would you recommend to reduce the risk of neonatal varicella infection?

a) Delay her induction for a week
b) Deliver by elective caesarean section
c) Intravenous aciclovir for the neonate
d) Intravenous aciclovir in labour
e) Oral aciclovir for the mother from diagnosis

Correct response: a

Explanation

Planned delivery should be delayed for at least seven days, to allow placental transfer of maternal antibodies.

Royal College of Obstetricians & Gynaecologists. *Chickenpox in Pregnancy*. Green-top Guideline No. 13, September 2007.

143

A 32-year-old primigravida is admitted in spontaneous labour with confirmed ruptured membranes at 39 weeks of gestation. Her temperature is 38.5 °C.

In this case, what is the estimated risk of early-onset neonatal group B streptococcal (EOGBS) disease?

a) 1/10
b) 1/20
c) 1/100
d) 1/200
e) 1/1000

Correct response: d

Explanation

Intrapartum pyrexia (> 38 °C) is associated with a risk of EOGBS disease of 5.3/1000 (versus a background risk of 0.5/1000). In view of this increased risk, intrapartum antibiotic prophylaxis for group B streptococcal disease should be offered in the presence of maternal pyrexia.

Royal College of Obstetricians & Gynaecologists. *The Prevention of Early-onset Neonatal Group B Streptococcal Disease*. Green-top Guideline No. 36, July 2012.

144

A 29-year-old woman is referred to the gynaecology clinic with a history of recurrent first-trimester miscarriages. Initial investigations were negative for anticardiolipin antibodies and lupus anticoagulant. She has no other medical problems. Previous cytogenetic analysis on products of conception showed normal fetal karyotype.

Which one of the following investigations should be recommended next?

a) Hysteroscopy
b) Inherited thrombophilia screen
c) LH/FSH ratio

d) Parental karyotyping
e) Ultrasound scan of pelvis

Correct response: e

Explanation
All women with first-trimester miscarriages should have a pelvic ultrasound scan to assess uterine anatomy. Hysteroscopy is required only if uterine anomaly is suspected. Inherited thrombophilia screen is not recommended for first-trimester miscarriages. Parental karyotyping is advised only when cytogenetic analysis of products reveals an unbalanced translocation. Luteinizing hormone (LH)/follicle-stimulating hormone (FSH) and androgen profile are of no proven value in the management of recurrent miscarriage.

Royal College of Obstetricians & Gynaecologists. *The Investigation and Treatment of Couples with Recurrent First-trimester and Second-trimester Miscarriage*. Green-top Guideline No. 17, April 2011.

145

A 29-year-old woman presents with a history of heavy vaginal bleeding two weeks after having a normal vaginal birth. Clinical assessment indicates retained products of conception, and she is consented for surgical evacuation of retained products of conception (ERPC).

What is the risk of uterine perforation in this case?

a) 1%
b) 5%
c) 10%
d) 15%
e) 20%

Correct response: b

Explanation
Studies report a range of incidence of uterine perforation. When surgical ERPC is carried out in the postpartum period, 5% of cases have been associated with uterine perforation.

Shakir F, Diab Y. The perforated uterus. *The Obstetrician & Gynaecologist* 2013; **15**: 256–61.

146

A woman is being treated with magnesium sulphate for severe pre-eclampsia. There is concern about magnesium toxicity.

What is the first sign of magnesium toxicity?

a) Bradycardia
b) Decreased urine output
c) Loss of deep tendon reflexes
d) Reduced consciousness
e) Respiratory depression

Correct response: c

Explanation

Reduced urine output causes increased magnesium levels due to decreased excretion. The first warning of impending toxicity is loss of the patellar reflex at plasma concentrations between 3.5 and 5 mmol/L. Respiratory paralysis occurs at 5–6.5 mmol/L. Cardiac conduction is altered at > 7.5 mmol/L, and cardiac arrest can be expected when concentrations of magnesium exceed 12.5 mmol/L.

Lu JF, Nightingale CH. Magnesium sulfate in eclampsia and pre-eclampsia: pharmacokinetic principles. *Clinical Pharmacokinetics* 2000; **38**: 305–14.

147

A couple presented with a history of primary infertility. The male partner has cystic fibrosis, and semen analysis showed azoospermia.

What is the most likely cause of azoospermia in this patient?

a) Congenital absence of ejaculatory duct
b) Congenital bilateral absence of seminal vesicles
c) Congenital bilateral absence of vas deferens
d) Obstruction following genitourinary infection
e) Retrograde ejaculation

Correct response: c

Explanation

Congenital bilateral absence of the vas deferens (CBAVD) is found in association with mutated cystic fibrosis transmembrane conductance regulator (*CFTR*) alleles.

National Institute for Health and Care Excellence (NICE). *Fertility: Assessment and Treatment for People with Fertility Problems.* NICE Clinical Guideline CG156, February 2013.

148

A 20-year-old woman has had side effects to various hormonal contraceptives. She is not keen on intrauterine devices. She wants to try a cervical cap with spermicide.

What is the optimum duration of application for a cervical cap for it to be most effective?

a) Insert just before intercourse and remove immediately
b) Insert just before intercourse and remove after 6 hours
c) Insert an hour before intercourse and remove an hour after
d) Insert an hour before intercourse and remove after 3 hours
e) Insert an hour before intercourse and remove after 12 hours

Correct response: b

Explanation

Although cervical caps are an uncommon form of contraception (less than 1% of women in a survey in 2008/09), they are an effective form of contraception for those who are prepared to accept a pregnancy rate of between 6% and 12%.

Faculty of Sexual & Reproductive Healthcare. *Clinical Guidance: Barrier Contraception and STI Prevention*, August 2012. http://www.fsrh.org/pdfs/CEUGuidanceBarrierMethodsAug12.pdf (accessed 17 November 2014).

149

A 25-year-old woman intending to commence the combined contraceptive pill wants to discuss the risk of venous thromboembolism (VTE). She has no other risk factors for VTE.

Which progestogen in combined oral contraceptives is associated with the lowest risk of VTE?

a) Desogestrel
b) Drospirenone
c) Etonogestrel
d) Gestodene
e) Norgestimate

Correct response: e

Explanation
A recent warning from the Medicines and Healthcare Products Regulatory Agency (MHRA) says that levonorgestrel, norgestimate and norethisterone have an incidence of 5–7 VTEs per 10 000 women per year of use against a background of 2. Etonogestrel and norelgestromin have a risk of 6–12, and for gestodene, desogestrel and drospirenone it is 9–12.

Faculty of Sexual & Reproductive Healthcare. *Statement: Venous Thromboembolism (VTE) and Hormonal Contraception*, November 2014. http://www.fsrh.org/pdfs/FSRHStatementVTEandHormonalContraception.pdf (accessed 17 November 2014).

150

A 25-year-old primiparous woman had a second-trimester miscarriage at 16 weeks. She had painless dilatation of cervix followed by rupture of membranes. There is no history of cervical surgery.

What is the most appropriate management for future pregnancy?

a) Abdominal cerclage pre-pregnancy
b) Cervical cerclage at 13–15 weeks
c) Clinical assessment of cervical length at 14 weeks
d) Pre-pregnancy assessment of cervical length
e) Serial sonographic surveillance of cervical length in pregnancy

Correct response: e

Explanation
History-indicated cerclage should be offered to women with three or more previous preterm births and/or second-trimester losses. For a woman with only one mid-trimester loss, serial sonographic surveillance of cervical length is recommended.

Royal College of Obstetricians & Gynaecologists. *The Investigation and Treatment of Couples with Recurrent First-trimester and Second-trimester Miscarriage*. Green-top Guideline No. 17, April 2011.

A ..-year-old primigravida is 33 weeks pregnant. She reports to the day assessment unit with a second episode of reduced fetal movements. Initial examination and cardiotocography (CTG) are normal.

What is the most appropriate next step?

a) Deliver baby following a course of steroids
b) Reassure her and provide her with a kick chart
c) Repeat CTG in 2 days
d) Ultrasound scan
e) Umbilical artery Doppler study

Correct response: d

Explanation
Perception of fetal movements is an important way to monitor a baby. If a woman is busy and on her feet, she will often not be aware of movements. If she is sitting she will be aware of more, and most movements are felt when lying down. Some women experience a reduction of fetal movements if prescribed steroids, and sedating drugs such as alcohol or opioids can reduce movements. Fetal presentation makes no difference to the perception of fetal movements, but women feel fewer movements when the fetal back is anterior. Women who present on two or more occasions with reduced fetal movements are almost twice as likely to have a poor perinatal outcome as those who present only once.

Royal College of Obstetricians & Gynaecologists. *Reduced Fetal Movements*. Green-top Guideline No. 57, February 2011.
Unterscheider J, Horgan R, O'Donoghue K, Greene R. Reduced fetal movements. *The Obstetrician & Gynaecologist* 2009; **11**: 245–51.

152

A 28-year-old in her first pregnancy has delivered normally and has had early cord clamping and 10 IU of oxytocin IM and controlled cord traction applied. The placenta has not delivered yet.

After how long would you call it a prolonged third stage of labour?

a) 10 minutes
b) 20 minutes
c) 30 minutes
d) 45 minutes
e) 60 minutes

Correct response: c

Explanation
In a physiological third stage, 60 minutes would be allowed. First-line management should be an injection of 20 IU oxytocin in 20 mL saline into the umbilical vein. Intravenous oxytocin is not recommended.

National Institute for Health and Care Excellence (NICE). *Intrapartum Care: Care of Healthy Women and Their Babies During Childbirth*. NICE Clinical Guideline CG55, September 2007.

153

A 16-year-old girl presents with primary amenorrhoea. She is examined have normal secondary sexual characteristics but a small blind-en Ultrasound scan reveals normal ovaries, and she has normal XX chro karyotyping.

What condition does this girl most likely have?

a) 5-Alpha-reductase type 2 deficiency
b) Complete androgen insensitivity syndrome
c) Congenital adrenal hyperplasia (CAH)
d) Mayer–Rokitansky–Küster–Hauser (MRKH) syndrome
e) Swyer's syndrome

Correct response: d

Explanation
MRKH syndrome occurs in 1 in 5000 births and is characterized by the absence of vagina, cervix and uterus, but normal ovaries. Congenital abnormalities of the urinary tract are common, occurring in about 40% of cases. 5-Alpha-reductase type 2 deficiency, androgen insensitivity syndrome and Swyer's syndrome would have XY chromosomes. The vagina is normal in CAH.

Luesley DM, Baker PN, eds. *Obstetrics and Gynaecology: an Evidence-based Text for MRCOG*, 2nd edition. London: E. Arnold, 2010.
Valappil S, Chetan U, Wood N, Garden A. Mayer–Rokitansky–Küster–Hauser syndrome: diagnosis and management. *The Obstetrician & Gynaecologist* 2012; 14: 93–8.

154

A 24-year-old woman presents to the emergency department with light vaginal bleeding after five weeks of amenorrhoea. A recent pregnancy test was positive. She also complains of sharp pain in the left iliac fossa. Blood tests reveal that she is O negative blood group.

Which subsequent outcome would require anti-D prophylaxis?

a) Complete miscarriage
b) Expectant management of early fetal demise
c) Medical management of ectopic pregnancy
d) Medical management of miscarriage
e) Surgical management of ectopic pregnancy

Correct response: e

Explanation
Anti-D prophylaxis is only required with surgical management of a miscarriage or ectopic pregnancy.

National Institute for Health and Care Excellence (NICE). *Ectopic Pregnancy and Miscarriage: Diagnosis and Initial Management in Early Pregnancy of Ectopic Pregnancy and Miscarriage*. NICE Clinical Guideline CG154, December 2012.

You are taking consent from a primigravida for an elective caesarean section for major placenta praevia. You explain that one of the serious risks associated with the procedure is massive obstetric haemorrhage.

Which of the following best represents the risk of massive obstetric haemorrhage in this woman?

a) 5 in 100
b) 10 in 100
c) 20 in 100
d) 30 in 100
e) 50 in 100

Correct response: c

Explanation
Overall, the risk of massive haemorrhage associated with caesarean section for placenta praevia is 12 times normal. Even without a previous caesarean section, women with placenta praevia have an increased risk of placenta accreta, which will increase the risk of haemorrhage.

Royal College of Obstetricians & Gynaecologists. *Caesarean Section for Placenta Praevia*. Consent Advice No. 12, December 2010.

156

A 28-year-old primigravida at 38 weeks of gestation presents with a history of rupture of membranes six hours ago. She is apyrexial, is not having any contractions, and is confirmed to be draining clear liquor. While writing your notes, you discover that she has been recently treated for a group B streptococcal urinary tract infection.

What should you offer her next?

a) Augmentation of labour and prophylactic intravenous antibiotics in 24 hours
b) Augmentation of labour and prophylactic intravenous antibiotics immediately
c) Augmentation of labour immediately and intravenous antibiotics when contracting
d) Intravenous antibiotics with the onset of active labour
e) Prophylactic intravenous antibiotics immediately and await events

Correct response: b

Explanation
Group B *Streptococcus* (GBS; *Streptococcus agalactiae*) is recognized as the most frequent cause of severe early-onset (< 7 days of age) infection in newborn infants. Screening for GBS carriage is routinely performed in the USA and Canada. This is not the practice in the UK. Despite this, the prevalence of early-onset group B streptococcal (EOGBS) disease in the UK is 0.5/1000 births, very similar to that in the USA. Intrapartum antibiotic prophylaxis reduces the incidence of early-onset disease but has no effect on late-onset (> 7 days) disease. Intrapartum antibiotic prophylaxis in the form of benzylpenicillin or clindamycin should be given as soon as possible after the onset of labour.

Royal College of Obstetricians & Gynaecologists. *The Prevention of Early-onset Neonatal Group B Streptococcal Disease*. Green-top Guideline No. 36, July 2012.

157

You are teaching a midwife how to perform McRoberts' manoeuvre.

Which of the following best describes McRoberts' manoeuvre?

a) Extension and abduction of maternal hips
b) Extension and adduction of maternal hips
c) Flexion and abduction of maternal hips
d) Flexion and abduction of maternal knees
e) Flexion and adduction of maternal hips

Correct response: c

Explanation
Shoulder dystocia occurs when either the anterior or, less commonly, the posterior fetal shoulder impacts on the maternal symphysis or sacral promontory, respectively. Additional obstetric manoeuvres are required to deliver the fetus after the head has delivered and gentle traction has failed. An understanding of each of these manoeuvres is essential to ensure that the best care can be given to the mother and baby in this life-threatening situation. The ability to teach trainees, midwives and students is part of a practising obstetrician's role.

Royal College of Obstetricians & Gynaecologists. *Shoulder Dystocia*, 2nd edition. Green-top Guideline No. 42, July 2012.

158

A 25-year-old man was referred with a history of secondary subfertility. Semen analysis confirmed azoospermia on two separate occasions two months apart. His initial hormone profile indicated reduced follicle-stimulating hormone (FSH) (0.6 IU/L) and luteinizing hormone (LH) (0.8 IU/L) concentrations.

What condition is the most likely explanation?

a) Cystic fibrosis carrier
b) Klinefelter syndrome
c) Taking anabolic steroids
d) Taking azathioprine
e) Varicocele

Correct response: c

Explanation
Low FSH and LH concentrations suggest hypogonadotrophic hypogonadism. A male cystic fibrosis carrier might have azoospermia due to congenital bilateral absence of the vas deferens, but with normal FSH and LH levels. A man with Klinefelter syndrome would have primary testicular failure with elevated FSH and LH concentrations. In both conditions, the man would not able to father a child naturally. Azathioprine does not have any effect on spermatogenesis. It is doubtful whether varicoceles have any negative impact on male subfertility or spermatogenesis. Anabolic steroids exert a negative effect on the hypothalamic–pituitary–testicular axis, resulting in hypogonadotrophic hypogonadism.

Dejaco C, Mittermaier C, Reinisch W, *et al*. Azathioprine treatment and male fertility in inflammatory bowel disease. *Gastroenterology* 2001; **121**: 1048–53.

Karavolos S, Stewart J, Evbuomwan I, McEleny K, Aird I. Assessment of the infertile male. *The Obstetrician & Gynaecologist* 2013; **15**: 1–9.

159

A 25-year-old woman attends your clinic for review. She presents with three unexplained first-trimester miscarriages.

What is the estimated miscarriage rate in her next pregnancy?

a) 20%
b) 30%
c) 40%
d) 50%
e) 60%

Correct response: b

Explanation

The risk of a further miscarriage increases with the number of miscarriages, with a 53% chance of further miscarriage after six or more miscarriages. The prognosis is not poor, with a 1994 study showing that over 66% of women with unexplained miscarriages attending a recurrent miscarriage clinic had a full-term pregnancy.

Clifford K, Rai R, Regan L. Future pregnancy outcome in unexplained recurrent first trimester miscarriage. *Human Reproduction* 1997; **12**: 387–9.
Morley L, Shillito J, Tang T. Preventing recurrent miscarriage of unknown aetiology. *The Obstetrician & Gynaecologist* 2013; **15**: 99–105.

160

You are teaching a group of medical students on maternal obesity. They would like to know the impact of obesity on pregnant women.

As reported by the Centre for Maternal and Child Enquiries (CMACE) for the years 2006–08, what percentage of maternal deaths involved women who were obese?

a) 5–10%
b) 11–15%
c) 16–20%
d) 21–25%
e) 26–30%

Correct response: e

Explanation

The correct answer is 27%. Obese women are overrepresented in the direct as opposed to the indirect deaths. During pregnancy, obese women are at increased risk of several adverse perinatal outcomes, including anaesthetic, perioperative and other maternal and fetal complications. They have higher rates of induction, failed induction and caesarean section. Caesarean section rates in nulliparous women are 20.7% in normal-weight women, rising to 27.5% in obese women and 47.4% in the morbidly obese. This will influence the highest cause of death for obese women, which is thromboembolism. Seventy-eight per cent of the women who died in 2006–08 from thromboembolism were overweight or obese. In other categories, weight was a factor in cardiac disease (61% overweight or obese) but was not a factor in suicide, haemorrhage or sepsis, where the rates were around the national average (20–25%). For other causes, weight contributed to death, with around 40% of obese women in each category. A study of the most morbidly obese women (body mass index > 50) by the UK Obstetric Surveillance System (UKOSS) in 2007–08 showed that they were at increased risk of pre-eclampsia, gestational diabetes, admission to ICU, caesarean section and general anaesthesia.

Centre for Maternal and Child Enquiries (CMACE). *Maternal Obesity in the UK: Findings from a National Project*. London: CMACE, 2010.

Centre for Maternal and Child Enquiries (CMACE). Saving mothers' lives: reviewing maternal deaths to make motherhood safer: 2006–2008. The Eighth Report of the Confidential Enquiries into Maternal Deaths in the United Kingdom. *BJOG* 2011; **118** (Suppl. 1): 1–203.

Stewart FM, Ramsay JE, Greer IA. Obesity: impact on obstetric practice and outcome. *The Obstetrician & Gynaecologist* 2009; **11**: 25–31.

161

A 22-year-old woman attends her postnatal review six weeks after the delivery of her first child. She has had an emergency caesarean section at 33 weeks of gestation for severe pre-eclampsia complicated with HELLP syndrome.

What is her risk of developing pre-eclampsia in her next pregnancy?

a) 1 in 2
b) 1 in 4
c) 1 in 6
d) 1 in 8
e) 1 in 10

Correct response: b

Explanation

Women who have pre-eclampsia are at significant risk of developing gestational hypertension in a subsequent pregnancy. The earlier and more serious their symptoms, the more likely it is that they will have future problems. Gestational hypertension is as high as 1 in 2, and pre-eclampsia ranges from a 16% risk with mild pre-eclampsia to 25% as in this case, to 55% if the woman delivered before 28 weeks.

National Institute for Health and Care Excellence (NICE). *Hypertension in Pregnancy: the Management of Hypertensive Disorders during Pregnancy*. NICE Clinical Guideline CG107, August 2010.

162

A woman known to be a group B *Streptococcus* (GBS) carrier in her current pregnancy presents with a history of rupture of membranes at 33 weeks of gestation. She is well and is not in established labour. Her previous child was admitted to the neonatal unit and treated with antibiotics for confirmed neonatal GBS infection at birth.

What is the most appropriate next step in her management, once you have confirmed rupture of membranes?

a) Administer steroids and observe
b) Administer steroids, commence intravenous benzylpenicillin and induce labour in 24 hours
c) Administer steroids, commence intravenous benzylpenicillin and observe

d) Administer steroids, commence oral erythromycin and induce labour in 24 hours
e) Administer steroids, commence oral erythromycin and observe

Correct response: e

Explanation
The risk of delivery outweighs the risk of infection. The woman should be treated as any other woman presenting with preterm premature rupture of the membranes.

Royal College of Obstetricians & Gynaecologists. *The Prevention of Early-onset Neonatal Group B Streptococcal Disease.* Green-top Guideline No. 36, July 2012.

163

You are counselling a primigravida with a breech presentation at 37 weeks of gestation for external cephalic version (ECV).

What is the rate of spontaneous version in this woman if ECV is not performed?

a) 2%
b) 5%
c) 8%
d) 11%
e) 14%

Correct response: c

Explanation
Women should be offered ECV. Although spontaneous version may occur, ECV at term reduces the incidence of non-cephalic presentation at delivery (RR 0.38, 95% CI 0.18–0.80, risk difference 52%, NNT 2). Spontaneous version rates for nulliparous women are approximately 8% after 36 weeks but less than 5% after unsuccessful ECV; success rates of ECV are 30–80%. Spontaneous reversion to breech presentation after successful ECV occurs in less than 5%.

Royal College of Obstetricians & Gynaecologists. *External Cephalic Version and Reducing the Incidence of Breech Presentation.* Green-top Guideline No. 20a, December 2006.
Royal College of Obstetricians & Gynaecologists. *Caesarean Section for Placenta Praevia.* Consent Advice No. 12, December 2010.

164

A 38-year-old woman attends your antenatal clinic. She is known to carry monochorionic twins. At 28 weeks, one of the twins unfortunately dies in utero. The woman wants to know the risk of death of the surviving twin in the event of the pregnancy continuing.

What is the risk of death of the co-twin?

a) 12%
b) 22%
c) 32%
d) 42%
e) 52%

Correct response: a

Explanation
The risk of perinatal mortality is high in monochorionic twins even when both survive beyond 28 weeks, and is quoted as 3.3%. The perinatal mortality rate up to 24 weeks is 11–14%.

Ong SS, Zamora J, Khan KS, Kilby MD. Prognosis for the co-twin following single-twin death: a systematic review. *BJOG* 2006; **113**: 992–8.

Royal College of Obstetricians & Gynaecologists. *Management of Monochorionic Twin Pregnancy*. Green-top Guideline No. 51, December 2008.

165

The midwife in the clinic shows you a blood result of a woman booked under you. The result shows she has anti-D antibodies. She is 24 weeks into her second pregnancy. The first was a term birth and the baby was well.

What titre of anti-D level would prompt you to refer the patient to a fetal medicine specialist?

a) Anti-D levels: 0.5 IU/mL
b) Anti-D levels: 1.5 IU/mL
c) Anti-D levels: 2.5 IU/mL
d) Anti-D levels: 3.5 IU/mL
e) Anti-D levels: 4.5 IU/mL

Correct response: e

Explanation
Although rhesus iso-immunization is rare in practice today following the prophylactic use of anti-D, it is important to be aware that a woman may become sensitized during pregnancy.

Royal College of Obstetricians & Gynaecologists. *The Management of Women with Red Cell Antibodies during Pregnancy*. Green-top Guideline No. 65, May 2014.

166

A 60-year-old woman presents to your gynaecology clinic with a history of recurrent urinary tract infection (UTI) and symptoms of utero-vaginal prolapse.

Which of the following is a description of recurrent UTI?

a) At least two UTIs over a 12-month period
b) At least three UTIs over a 12-month period
c) At least four UTIs over a 12-month period
d) At least five UTIs over a 12-month period
e) At least six UTIs over a 12-month period

Correct response: b

Explanation
Recurrent UTI may be related to a prolapse if it leads to significant residual urine. If this is not the case, surgery is unlikely to make any difference.

Royal College of Obstetricians & Gynaecologists. StratOG eLearning. https://stratog.rcog.org.uk (accessed 17 November 2014).

167

A 15-year-old girl presents with primary amenorrhoea although her secondary sexual characteristics are normally developed. She complains of having cyclical lower abdominal pain over the previous six months.

What is the most likely diagnosis?

a) Androgen insensitivity syndrome
b) Constitutional delay
c) Hyperprolactinaemia
d) Imperforate hymen
e) Pregnancy

Correct response: d

Explanation

An imperforate hymen or transverse vaginal septum often presents with cyclical abdominal pain. Women with androgen insensitivity syndrome will have scanty pubic hair, since there is no androgen response in target tissues.

Royal College of Obstetricians & Gynaecologists. StratOG eLearning. https://stratog.rcog.org.uk (accessed 17 November 2014).

168

A 28-year-old nulliparous woman presents to your gynaecology clinic with a history of infrequent periods occurring every three to four months since menarche at 13. Her body mass index (BMI) is 32. She suffers from mild asthma and has no other medical or surgical history of note.

What is the most likely cause for her presentation?

a) Excessive physical exercise
b) Hyperthyroidism
c) Ovarian cysts
d) Polycystic ovary syndrome
e) Prolactinoma

Correct response: d

Explanation

Polycystic ovary syndrome is very common and is often associated with obesity.

Royal College of Obstetricians & Gynaecologists. StratOG eLearning. https://stratog.rcog.org.uk (accessed 17 November 2014).

169

A woman had a difficult abdominal hysterectomy for a fibroid uterus. The transverse suprapubic incision needed to be extended laterally on both sides to facilitate the surgery. Postoperatively she developed sharp, burning pain and paraesthesia over her mons pubis, labia and the lateral aspect of her thigh. On examination, no motor weakness is found.

Which nerve is affected?

a) Femoral
b) Genitofemoral
c) Ilioinguinal
d) Lateral cutaneous nerve of the thigh
e) Obturator

Correct response: c

Explanation

The injury to this nerve is typically caused by nerve entrapment at the lateral borders of the incision, especially when the incision is extended beyond the lateral border of the rectus abdominis muscle.

Kuponiyi O, Alleemudder DI, Latunde-Dada A, Eadarapalli P. Nerve injuries associated with gynaecological surgery. *The Obstetrician & Gynaecologist* 2014; 16: 29–36.

170

An 89-year-old woman is reviewed in the urogynaecology clinic. She complains of increased frequency of urination, urgency, urge incontinence and nocturia. Her symptoms are disturbing her quality of life. She is very frail and does not wish to have any surgical intervention.

Which of the following is the most appropriate first-line treatment for the management of her symptoms?

a) Duloxetine
b) Mirabegron
c) Oxybutynin
d) Solifenacin
e) Tolterodine

Correct response: e

Explanation

This woman's symptoms suggest an overactive bladder. NICE guideline CG171 recommends using oxybutynin, tolterodine or darifenacin as a first-line treatment in symptoms of overactive bladder. Oxybutynin should not be offered to frail older patients, since it crosses the blood–brain barrier and can lead to cognitive impairment.

National Institute for Health and Care Excellence (NICE). *Urinary Incontinence: the Management of Urinary Incontinence in Women.* NICE Clinical Guideline CG171, September 2013.

171

A 39-year-old woman is booked at 10 weeks of gestation in her second pregnancy. She was referred to a consultant-led antenatal clinic, because her booking blood test detected anti-c antibodies at a titre of 5.4 IU/mL.

What is the most appropriate antenatal management plan for this woman with regard to anti-c antibodies?

a) Anti-c levels should be measured every 4 weeks until delivery
b) Anti-c levels should be measured every 4 weeks up to 28 weeks of gestation and then every 2 weeks until delivery
c) Anti-c levels should be measured every 6 weeks up to 34 weeks of gestation and then every 2 weeks until delivery
d) Monitoring of anti-c levels is indicated only when anti-c levels are > 7.5 IU/mL at booking
e) Referral to a fetal medicine specialist is indicated, as anti-c titres do not correlate well with either the development or the severity of fetal anaemia

Correct response: b

Explanation
At least 40 red cell antigens are associated with haemolytic disease of the newborn. It is possible to test the woman's partner to assess if he is heterozygous, and in future, by harvesting fetal cells from the maternal circulation, it may be possible to assess the fetus. In general, the absolute titre is less important than the detection of rising titres.

Royal College of Obstetricians & Gynaecologists. *The Management of Women with Red Cell Antibodies during Pregnancy*. Green-top Guideline No. 65, May 2014.

172

A 27-year-old woman with a history of spinal cord injury (SCI) attends a pre-conception clinic along with her husband. This clinic is run by an obstetrician specializing in SCI in pregnancy. A care plan is discussed with this couple, based on the woman's disability and available support. The consultant informs them about autonomic dysreflexia, which is a potentially dangerous medical emergency in such cases.

Autonomic dysreflexia may develop in individuals with a neurological level of spinal cord injury:

a) Above the second lumbar vertebral level (L2)
b) At or above the fourth thoracic vertebral level (T4)
c) At or above the sixth thoracic vertebral level (T6)
d) At or above the twelfth thoracic vertebral level (T12)
e) Below the tenth thoracic vertebral level (T10)

Correct response: c

Explanation
Women with SCI usually find that pregnancy exacerbates their symptoms. Women with lesions above T6 are at risk of autonomic dysreflexia, spasms, breathing problems related to the growing fetus, bradycardia and hypotension. They are also at increased risk of pressure ulcers, urinary tract infections and chest infections. Women with a lesion above T10 will not be aware of the onset of labour. Autonomic dysreflexia is an emergency. Because of loss of control of the sympathetic outflow, something as minimal as fetal movements can lead to a rise in blood pressure. This stimulates the vagus nerve via baroreceptors and can lead to a life-threatening bradycardia. An epidural in labour is recommended to try to reduce the risk.

Dawood R, Altanis E, Ribes-Pastor P, Ashworth F. Pregnancy and spinal cord injury. *The Obstetrician & Gynaecologist* 2014; **16**: 99–107.

173

The consultant is asked to review a woman at 22 weeks of gestation, as her ultrasound scan suggests that the fetus has an echogenic bowel. The results of cytomegalovirus (CMV) tests performed two weeks previously indicate that she seroconverted in the previous three months. The samples were tested in parallel at the regional laboratory.

What is the risk of vertical transmission of CMV?

a) 10%
b) 20%
c) 30%
d) 40%
e) 50%

Correct response: d

Explanation

There is a 40% risk of vertical transmission in the first and second trimester, rising to 65% in the third trimester. The classical ultrasound picture shows bilateral periventricular calcification. Most neonates are initially asymptomatic, and 10–15% will develop neurodevelopmental damage in the first three years of life.

To M, Kidd M, Maxwell D. Prenatal diagnosis and management of fetal infections. *The Obstetrician & Gynaecologist* 2009; **11**: 108–16.

174

A primigravida presents at 33 weeks of gestation with a history of itching involving the palms and soles of the feet for one week. On examination, she has evidence of dermatographia artefacta. Her liver functions show modest elevation of both aspartate transaminase (AST) and alanine transaminase (ALT), and a normal bilirubin. There is no evidence of a rash.

What is the most likely clinical diagnosis?

a) Atopic eruption of pregnancy
b) Chronic active hepatitis
c) Pemphigoid gestationis
d) Obstetric cholestasis
e) Polymorphic eruption of pregnancy

Correct response: d

Explanation

Dermatographia artefacta is skin trauma from scratching due to the pruritis of obstetric cholestasis. It is important to differentiate it from other common skin conditions such as eczema or atopic eruption of pregnancy. If a rash is present, this may be polymorphic eruption of pregnancy or pemphigoid gestationis. Pruritis in pregnancy is common, affecting about a quarter of all pregnancies. The itching of obstetric cholestasis is typically worse at night, it may be widespread, and it typically includes the hands and soles of the feet.

Royal College of Obstetricians & Gynaecologists. *Obstetric Cholestasis*. Green-top Guideline No. 43, April 2011.

175

A woman at 28 weeks of gestation has been in contact with her neighbour who developed chickenpox two days ago. She is unclear about a previous history of chickenpox in childhood and visits her general practitioner.

What is the most appropriate next step?

a) Administer varicella-zoster immunoglobulin (VZIG)
b) Administer VZIG + varicella vaccine
c) Administer varicella vaccine
d) Reassure and discharge in the absence of a rash
e) Test her booking bloods for IgG antibodies to varicella

Correct response: e

Explanation

Since VZIG is effective up to 10 days after contact, best practice is to take blood to test for varicella-zoster virus (VZV) immunity.

Royal College of Obstetricians & Gynaecologists. *Chickenpox in Pregnancy*. Green-top Guideline No. 13, September 2007.

176

A woman presents at 36 weeks of gestation with a history of a previous caesarean section. Her previous baby was affected by early-onset group B *Streptococcus* (GBS). She is keen to deliver vaginally. She has been assessed by a consultant obstetrician and is suitable for a vaginal delivery. Her vaginal swab at 36 weeks is negative for GBS.

What mode of delivery is best suited for her, considering her history?

a) Elective caesarean section at 39 + 0 with antibiotic prophylaxis against GBS
b) Elective caesarean section at 39 + 0 with routine surgical antibiotic prophylaxis
c) Vaginal delivery with antibiotic prophylaxis against GBS in active labour
d) Vaginal delivery with routine measures and assessment of the baby for infection at birth
e) Vaginal delivery with routine measures, as the swab in this pregnancy is negative

Correct response: c

Explanation

Antibiotic prophylaxis is advised for all women with a previously affected baby, even when the swab has been negative in the current pregnancy.

Royal College of Obstetricians & Gynaecologists. *The Prevention of Early-onset Neonatal Group B Streptococcal Disease*. Green-top Guideline No. 36, July 2012.

177

A primigravid woman is in spontaneous labour at term with an effective epidural anaesthesia. She has been in the second stage of labour for three hours with regular contractions 4 in 10. The head is not palpable per abdomen. The last vaginal examination confirmed the cervix is fully dilated, vertex presenting, station at the spines and right occiput posterior (ROP) position. The cardiotocogram (CTG) is reassuring. She has now been actively pushing for two hours.

What would be your immediate course of action?

a) Allow another hour of pushing
b) Caesarean section, category 2
c) Direct traction forceps in theatre
d) Instrumental delivery with ventouse with an occipito-posterior (OP) cup in theatre
e) Instrumental delivery with silastic cup in delivery suite room

Correct response: d

Explanation
The National Institute for Health and Care Excellence (NICE) recommends referral for an operative delivery if birth is not imminent after two hours of active pushing in a primiparous woman and one hour in a multiparous woman.

National Institute for Health and Care Excellence (NICE). *Intrapartum Care: Care of Healthy Women and Their Babies During Childbirth*. NICE Clinical Guideline CG55, September 2007.

Royal College of Obstetricians & Gynaecologists. *Operative Vaginal Delivery*. Green-top Guideline No. 26, January 2011.

178

A woman who is para 5 has polyhydramnios and pre-eclampsia. She has previously had five normal vaginal deliveries. Her progress of labour has been good with an active phase of labour lasting six hours. Delivery is now imminent.

What is the most appropriate immediate postpartum management?

a) Misoprostol 1000 µg PR post delivery
b) Oxytocin infusion 40 units at 125 mL/h post delivery
c) Oxytocin infusion 40 units at 125 mL/h + misoprostol 1000 µg PR post delivery
d) Syntometrine IM post delivery
e) 10 IU oxytocin IM post delivery

Correct response: e

Explanation
Active management of the third stage of labour with oxytocin reduces the risk of postpartum haemorrhage by 60%. Grand multiparous women are at risk of a primary postpartum haemorrhage so should be given a higher (10 IU) dose. Syntometrine has significant side effects and is only marginally better at reducing the risk of postpartum haemorrhage than oxytocin. Misoprostol is not as effective as oxytocin.

National Institute for Health and Care Excellence (NICE). *Intrapartum Care: Care of Healthy Women and Their Babies During Childbirth*. NICE Clinical Guideline CG55, September 2007 (section 1.8).

Royal College of Obstetricians & Gynaecologists. *Prevention and Management of Postpartum Haemorrhage*. Green-top Guideline No. 52, May 2009.

179

Uterine perforation is a complication of uterine manipulation that can cause severe morbidity and even mortality.

Which of the following procedures is associated with the highest risk of uterine perforation?

a) Evacuation of retained products of conception (ERPC) for postpartum haemorrhage
b) Hysteroscopy following endometrial ablation
c) Hysteroscopy for postmenopausal bleeding
d) Surgical termination of pregnancy (STOP)
e) Uterine manipulation at laparoscopy

Correct response: a

Explanation

The incidence of perforation after STOP is approximately 1/10 000. This is performed much more frequently than postpartum ERPC. It has been reported that the risk of perforation in postpartum evacuation is approximately 5%.

Shakir F, Diab Y. The perforated uterus. *The Obstetrician & Gynaecologist* 2013; **15**: 256–61.

180

A woman has undergone genetic testing for *BRCA1* and *BRCA2* gene carriage and has been told she is a carrier for the *BRCA1* gene, with a relative risk of developing ovarian cancer of 5. She asks you to explain relative risk to her.

Which one of the following best describes relative risk?

a) The difference in risk of a particular condition between those who are affected and those who are not
b) The number of people who must be treated to result in benefit to one person
c) The odds of an event happening in the affected group, expressed as a proportion of the odds of an event happening in the unaffected group
d) The rate of disease in the affected group divided by the rate of disease in the control group multiplied by the usual rate of the disease in the unaffected group
e) The rate of disease in the affected group divided by the rate of disease in the unaffected group

Correct response: e

Explanation

(a) = attributable risk
(b) = number needed to treat (NNT)
(c) = odds ratio (OR)
(d) = absolute risk

The ability to understand and critically appraise research papers, and to use the information to inform patients, is an essential skill in clinical practice.

British Menopause Society. Explaining risk and study design. BMS Fact Sheet. http://www.thebms.org.uk/factdetail.php?id=9 (accessed 17 November 2014).

181

A 30-year-old woman is referred to your gynaecology clinic having had a forceps delivery complicated by a haematoma four months previously. She is complaining of pain in the vulval, perineal and perianal region.

Which of the following would *not* support your diagnosis of pudendal neuralgia?

a) Pain much worse in the seated position
b) Pain radiates to anterior part of thigh
c) Reduced awareness of defecation
d) Sexual dysfunction
e) Urinary hesitancy and frequency

Correct response: b

Explanation

Pudendal neuralgia is a rare but disabling condition. It is more usually found following sacrospinous fixation or major pelvic surgery but can occur following nerve compression by a haematoma.

Possover M, Forman A. Neuropelveological assessment of neuropathic pelvic pain. *Gynecological Surgery* 2014; **11**: 139–44.

182

A 72-year-old woman who is generally fit and well is referred to you by the surgeons. She has been admitted with left iliac fossa pain, and an ultrasound scan has suggested that gynaecological review is warranted. Her ultrasound scan shows a small anteverted uterus with an endometrial thickness of 3 mm. The left ovary shows no obvious mass, while the right ovary contains a 3.2 × 4.2 × 4.9 mm simple cyst. There is no free fluid seen. Her CA-125 is 16 IU/mL.

How would you manage this woman?

a) Laparoscopic bilateral salpingo-oophorectomy
b) Laparoscopic oophorectomy
c) Refer for discussion at the multidisciplinary team meetings
d) Repeat ultrasound in 4 months
e) Ultrasound-guided aspiration of cyst

Correct response: d

Explanation

A simple small ovarian cyst will not be the cause of her pain. The risk of malignancy index (RMI) is 0 since the cyst is simple. RMI is calculated as CA-125 level multiplied by 1 if premenopausal or 3 if postmenopausal, multiplied by ultrasound findings of 0–3. If the cyst is simple with no solid areas or septations, it is 0. The risk of malignancy with a simple cyst is < 1%, and 50% of these cysts will resolve spontaneously within three months.

Royal College of Obstetricians & Gynaecologists. *Ovarian Cysts in Postmenopausal Women*. Green-top Guideline No. 34, October 2003, reviewed 2010.

183

During a vaginal repair, the assisting junior doctor asks about the different suture materials used. At that point, you are using polyglactin (Vicryl). You explain it is absorbable.

How long does it take to be absorbed?

a) 45–60 days
b) 60–90 days
c) 90–120 days
d) 120–180 days
e) 180–210 days

Correct response: b

Explanation

The choice of suture is important and relates to the tissue being sutured, the type of incision, the risk of infection and the frailty of the patient. Catgut is no longer used in the UK. Its tensile strength is poor and it causes a moderate tissue reaction. Most sutures used have a good tensile strength and low tissue reaction, and are absorbed in 60–120 days. These include polyglycolic acid (Dexon), polyglactic 910 (Vicryl) and polyglecaprone (Monocryl). For situations where additional support is required, polydioxanone (PDS) or polytrimethylene carbonate (Maxon) may be used. They will absorb in 180–210 days.

Raghavan R, Arya P, Arya P, China S. Abdominal incisions and sutures in obstetrics and gynaecology. *The Obstetrician & Gynaecologist* 2014; **16**: 13–18.

184

A medical student is attending colposcopy clinic with you, and asks you why the area you are looking at is called the transformation zone of the cervix.

Which of the following best describes the transformation zone of the cervix?

a) Glandular transformation of squamous epithelium
b) Metaplastic transformation of columnar to squamous epithelium
c) Pre-cancerous transformation of squamous epithelium
d) Transformation from columnar to transitional epithelium
e) Transformation from squamous to transitional epithelium

Correct response: b

Explanation

For a clinical educator, it is important to understand the basic physiology and anatomy that applies in clinical practice. This area of the cervix is vulnerable as it undergoes transformation from columnar to squamous epithelium and hence is commonly the site of premalignant and malignant disease.

Royal College of Obstetricians & Gynaecologists. StratOG eLearning. https://stratog.rcog.org.uk (accessed 17 November 2014).

185

A woman who is about to undergo an assisted vaginal delivery needs a pudendal nerve block as she has inadequate analgesia.

What are the three branches of the pudendal nerve?

a) Inferior rectal nerve, perineal nerve, dorsal nerve of the clitoris
b) Inferior rectal nerve, superior rectal nerve, perineal nerve
c) Perineal nerve, dorsal nerve of the clitoris, ilioinguinal nerve
d) Perineal nerve, ilioinguinal nerve, inferior gluteal nerve
e) Perineal nerve, inferior rectal nerve, superior gluteal nerve

Correct response: a

Explanation
It is important to be aware of the branches of the pudendal nerve, in order to understand the area that will be anaesthetized.

Ellis H, Mahadevan V. *Clinical Anatomy: Applied Anatomy for Students and Junior Doctors*, 12th edition. Chichester: Wiley, 2010.

186

A woman who is taking the combined oral contraceptive has been prescribed antibiotics by her general practitioner (GP). She attends the emergency gynaecology unit concerned about any need for barrier contraception, as her GP did not mention this.

Which drug is most likely to cause contraceptive failure?

a) Ciprofloxacin
b) Clindamycin
c) Erythromycin
d) Nitrofurantoin
e) Rifampicin

Correct response: e

Explanation
Many drugs alter the absorption, distribution, metabolism or excretion of oral contraceptive pills, which may increase or decrease serum concentrations and thus affect the reliability of the contraceptive. Clinicians need to be aware of this and counsel their patients accordingly.

Faculty of Sexual & Reproductive Healthcare. *Clinical Guidance: Drug Interactions with Hormonal Contraception*, January 2011. http://www.fsrh.org/pdfs/CEUguidance druginteractionshormonal.pdf (accessed 17 November 2014).

187

A 24-year-old woman is referred to the gynaecology clinic with a history of acne, hirsuitism and oligomenorrhoea. When you review the blood results, the testosterone is 8 nmol/L (normal < 1.5 nmol/L).

Which one of the following conditions would *not* be associated with a raised serum testosterone of 8 nmol/L?

a) Androgen-secreting tumour of the adrenal
b) Androgen-secreting tumour of the ovary
c) Congenital adrenal hyperplasia

d) Cushing's syndrome
e) Polycystic ovary syndrome

Correct response: e

Explanation
Polycystic ovary syndrome is a common condition, and the androgenic features are contributed to by the low levels of sex hormone binding globulin, which increases the free androgen index. Actual testosterone levels are usually only mildly raised, less than 5 nmol/L. Any testosterone level greater than 7 nmol/L should prompt investigation for another cause.

Meek CL, Bravis V, Don A, Kaplan F. Polycystic ovary syndrome and the differential diagnosis of hyperandrogenism. *The Obstetrician & Gynaecologist* 2013; **15**: 171–6.

188

A 34-year-old woman is 20 weeks in her first pregnancy. Her anomaly scan shows truncus arteriosus. She accepts your offer of amniocentesis.

Which investigation on amniotic fluid is most likely to identify the underlying cause?

a) Array comparative genomic hybridization (CGH)
b) Fluorescence in-situ hybridization (FISH) for 7q11 deletion (Williams syndrome)
c) G-banded karyotyping
d) Multiplex ligation-dependent probe amplification (MLPA) for subtelomeric rearrangements
e) Quantitative fluorescence polymerase chain reaction (QF-PCR) for common trisomies

Correct response: a

Explanation
Array CGH has much better resolution than standard karyotyping and will detect small chromosome deletions and duplications. 22q11 deletion is the most common syndromic cause of truncus arteriosus. Array CGH will detect this and other causes (including Williams syndrome).

Hillman S, McMullan DJ, Maher ER, Kilby MD. The use of chromosomal microarray in prenatal diagnosis. *The Obstetrician & Gynaecologist* 2013; **15**: 80–4.

189

A pregnant woman with a body mass index (BMI) of 35 undergoes oral glucose tolerance testing (OGTT) at 24 weeks of gestation. A standard 75 g OGTT is performed.

According to World Health Organization (WHO) criteria, what results confirm a diagnosis of gestational diabetes?

a) Fasting glucose of 5.8 mmol/L
b) One-hour glucose of 6.1 mmol/L
c) One-hour glucose of 7.8 mmol/L
d) Two-hour glucose of 7.6 mmol/L
e) Two-hour glucose of 7.9 mmol/L

Correct response: e

Explanation
One-hour values are not part of 75 g OGTT. Fasting glucose should be less than 6.1 mmol/L, and two-hour glucose less than 7.8 mmol/L.

National Institute for Health and Care Excellence (NICE). *Diabetes in Pregnancy: Management of Diabetes and its Complications from Pre-Conception to the Postnatal Period*. NICE Clinical Guideline CG63, March 2008.

190

Basic neonatal resuscitation is life-saving, training is simple and feasible, and the cost is low.

Neonatal resuscitation training packages for traditional birth attendants have been shown in both randomized and non-randomized trials to reduce perinatal and neonatal deaths by:

a) 0–20%
b) 20–40%
c) 40–60%
d) 60–80%
e) > 80%

Correct response: b

Explanation
The UN's Millennium Development Goal (MDG) 4 sets targets to reduce the number of deaths in children aged < 5 years by 2015. Basic resuscitation is one area where action is required, and it should be part of mandatory training for staff on the labour ward.

Smith AC, Mutangiri W, Fox R, Crofts JF. Millennium Development Goal 4: reducing perinatal and neonatal mortality in low-resource settings. *The Obstetrician & Gynaecologist* 2014: **16**: 1–5.

191

A 26-year-old known HIV-positive woman on highly active antiretroviral therapy (HAART) presents at 38 + 3 weeks to the obstetric assessment unit with confirmed pre-labour spontaneous rupture of membranes. Review of her blood tests taken at 36 weeks of gestation reveals a CD4 count of 300 cells/picolitre and an undetectable viral load. Her first child was born by spontaneous vaginal delivery in the Democratic Republic of the Congo three years previously.

Following British HIV Association (BHIVA) guidance, what should her management plan be?

a) Admit for induction of labour
b) Allow 24 hours for the onset of spontaneous labour
c) Await the onset of spontaneous labour but perform caesarean section if not delivered within 12 hours
d) Deliver by caesarean section once a course of intramuscular steroids is complete
e) Deliver by caesarean section immediately

Correct response: a

Explanation

Pregnant women with an undetectable viral load at 36 weeks can be managed as per HIV-negative women with the exception of spontaneous rupture of membranes at term, when labour should be expedited.

British HIV Association guidelines for the management of HIV infection in pregnant women 2012. *HIV Medicine* 2012; **13** (Suppl. 2): 87–157. http://www.bhiva.org/documents/Guidelines/Pregnancy/2012/hiv1030_6.pdf (accessed 17 November 2014).

192

A 24-year-old primiparous woman with an uncomplicated monochorionic diamniotic twin pregnancy attends your antenatal clinic at 34 weeks of gestation requesting a plan regarding the timing of her delivery. On ultrasound scan, both babies are cephalic presentation.

What is the most appropriate advice?

a) Await spontaneous onset of labour
b) Elective caesarean section at 36 weeks of gestation following intramuscular steroid administration
c) Elective caesarean section at 39 weeks of gestation
d) Induction of labour at 36 weeks of gestation following intramuscular steroid administration
e) Induction of labour at 38 weeks of gestation

Correct response: d

Explanation

Monochorionic twins have an increased risk of fetal death if the pregnancy goes beyond 38 weeks of gestation, even in uncomplicated cases. If delivery is planned before 37 weeks, it is essential that steroids are given to reduce the incidence of respiratory distress. In uncomplicated dichorionic twins, offer delivery at 37 weeks of gestation.

National Institute for Health and Care Excellence (NICE). *Multiple Pregnancy: the Management of Twin and Triplet Pregnancies in the Antenatal Period.* NICE Clinical Guideline CG129, September 2011.

193

A 34-year-old woman had a total abdominal hysterectomy for chronic menorrhagia following unsuccessful endometrial ablation. Postoperatively, she complains of weakness of the left leg, along with paraesthesia over the anterior and medial thigh.

What is the most likely injury causing her symptoms?

a) Injury to femoral nerve
b) Injury to ilioinguinal and hypogastric nerves
c) Injury to lateral cutaneous nerve
d) Injury to obturator nerve
e) Injury to sciatic and common peroneal nerve

Correct response: a

Explanation
Abdominal hysterectomy is mostly responsible for this. In reports of gynaecological-associated neuropathy, the femoral nerve is most frequently implicated, with an incidence of at least 11%. Femoral neuropathy commonly occurs as a result of compression of the nerve against the pelvic sidewall as it emerges from the lateral border of the psoas muscle. This happens when excessively deep retractor blades are used, or during the lateral placement of retractors.

Kuponiyi O, Alleemudder DI, Latunde-Dada A, Eadarapalli P. Nerve injuries associated with gynaecological surgery. *The Obstetrician & Gynaecologist* 2014; **16**: 29–36.

194

A 36-year-old woman was noted to have a blood pressure of 160/100 mmHg three days after a normal vaginal delivery at 38 weeks of gestation. She was offered induction of labour following diagnosis of pre-eclampsia at 37 weeks + 3 days. She is an asthmatic and uses inhalers. Her latest blood results are haemoglobin 105 g/L (normal 115–165), platelets 180 × 10^9/L (normal 150–400), creatinine 100 µmol/L (normal 53–97), alanine transaminase (ALT) 35 IU/L (normal 5–40). She is not breastfeeding.

What is the most appropriate antihypertensive for this woman?

a) Bendroflumethiazide
b) Labetalol
c) Methyldopa
d) Nifedepine
e) Ramipril

Correct response: d

Explanation
Avoid labetalol because she is asthmatic, and ACE inhibitors because of her raised creatinine.

Smith M, Waugh J, Nelson-Piercy C. Management of postpartum hypertension. *The Obstetrician & Gynaecologist* 2013; **15**: 45–50.

195

A 20-year-old woman presents to the emergency department with a short history of feeling unwell, fever and rigor two days after a vaginal delivery. Her pulse rate is 120 bpm, blood pressure 80/50 mmHg, temperature 38.5 °C, urine dipstick clear. An offensive lochia was noted on examination and vaginal swabs were taken. Full blood count revealed a white cell count of 23 × 10^9/L (normal 4–11), C-reactive protein 150 mg/L (normal < 10). An arterial blood gas showed lactate of 4 mmol/L (normal 0.5–2.2).

What should the next step in her investigation be?

a) Blood culture
b) Chest x-ray
c) Pelvic ultrasound
d) MRSA swabs
e) Urine culture

Correct response: a

Explanation
This patient is septic and requires immediate blood cultures so that intravenous antibiotics can be started. Genital tract sepsis is a major cause of maternal morbidity and mortality. The incidence of group A streptococcal (GAS) disease is about 1 per 10 000 live births (0.06/1000), and in the maternal mortality report *Saving mothers' lives* (2011) there were 26 deaths caused directly by maternal sepsis, with 13 due to GAS puerperal sepsis.

Palaniappan N, Menezes M, Willson P. Group A streptococcal puerperal sepsis: management and prevention. *The Obstetrician & Gynaecologist* 2012; **14**: 9–16.

Centre for Maternal and Child Enquiries (CMACE). Saving mothers' lives: reviewing maternal deaths to make motherhood safer: 2006–2008. The Eighth Report of the Confidential Enquiries into Maternal Deaths in the United Kingdom. *BJOG* 2011; **118** (Suppl. 1): 1–203.

196

A 34-year-old woman with known HIV on highly active antiretroviral treatment (HAART) comes to the labour ward at 37 weeks of gestation with pre-labour spontaneous rupture of membranes. She had a plasma viral load of < 50 copies/mL at 36 weeks. She has no other obstetric complications.

What is the most appropriate mode of delivery?

a) Augmentation of labour at 24 hours
b) Await spontaneous labour
c) Caesarean section at 24 hours after steroid administration
d) Emergency caesarean section
e) Immediate augmentation of labour

Correct response: e

Explanation
She has no contraindication to vaginal delivery, and the duration from membrane rupture to delivery should be minimized. Invasive monitoring is contraindicated, to minimize mother-to-child transmission.

British HIV Association guidelines for the management of HIV infection in pregnant women 2012. *HIV Medicine* 2012; **13** (Suppl. 2): 87–157. http://www.bhiva.org/documents/Guidelines/Pregnancy/2012/hiv1030_6.pdf (accessed 17 November 2014).

197

A 25-year-old woman is seen on the postnatal ward complaining of feeling unwell with fever and rigors two days after a caesarean delivery. Her pulse rate is 120 bpm, blood pressure 80/50 mmHg, temperature 38.5 °C, urine dipstick clear. She is noted to have an offensive lochia. Investigations reveal a white cell count of 23×10^9/L (normal 4–11), C-reactive protein 150 mg/L (normal < 10). An arterial blood gas shows lactate of 4 mmol/L (normal 0.5–2.2). Examination of the scar reveals violet discoloration around the edges with small blisters.

What is the most likely infective organism?

a) Anaerobes
b) *Escherichia coli*
c) *Clostridium perfringens*

d) Group A *Streptococcus*
e) Group B *Streptococcus*

Correct response: d

Explanation
She is developing necrotizing fasciitis. This is a very serious life-threatening condition. With aggressive management the death rate is still 20%.

Palaniappan N, Menezes M, Willson P. Group A streptococcal puerperal sepsis: management and prevention. *The Obstetrician & Gynaecologist* 2012; **14**: 9–16.

198

A 65-year-old woman presents with a sensation of a vaginal lump. She had a total abdominal hysterectomy for heavy periods 30 years ago. Examination reveals a vault prolapse.

On the POPQ scoring system, which point corresponds to the vaginal vault?

a) Aa
b) Bp
c) C
d) D
e) Tvl

Correct response: c

Explanation
The vaginal vault or cervix corresponds to point C on the POPQ (pelvic organ prolapse quantification) system. There is no point D if the patient has had a total hysterectomy.

Royal College of Obstetricians & Gynaecologists. *The Management of Post Hysterectomy Vaginal Vault Prolapse*. Green-top Guideline No. 46, October 2007.

199

A 30-year-old woman in her first pregnancy is admitted in labour at 36 weeks of gestation. Vaginal examination showed the cervix to be 6 cm dilated. The membranes ruptured soon after with blood-stained amniotic fluid. Following this, the fetal heart pattern changed and was interpreted as a sinusoidal trace.

What is the most appropriate management?

a) Augmentation with oxytocin
b) Caesarean section
c) Fetal blood sampling
d) Kleihauer test
e) Ultrasound with Doppler

Correct response: b

Explanation
A sinusoidal trace is classically associated with fetal bleeding and vasa praevia.

Royal College of Obstetricians & Gynaecologists. *Placenta Praevia, Placenta Praevia Accreta and Vasa Praevia: Diagnosis and Management*. Green-top Guideline No. 27, January 2011.

200

A 34-year-old presented to the delivery suite with a history of a sudden gush of watery vaginal discharge. She is 30 weeks pregnant in her first pregnancy, which is uncomplicated. A vaginal speculum examination confirmed ruptured membranes with clear liquor draining. A scan confirmed cephalic presentation. She was asked to attend the day assessment clinic twice weekly.

Which investigation is most likely to identify chorioamnionitis?

a) Biophysical profile
b) Blood test for C-reactive protein
c) Cardiotocography
d) Full blood count
e) Vaginal swabs

Correct response: c

Explanation

Cardiotogography (CTG) is useful, and indeed fetal tachycardia is used in the definition of clinical chorioamnionitis.

Royal College of Obstetricians & Gynaecologists. *Preterm Prelabour Rupture of Membranes*. Green-top Guideline No. 44, November 2006, amended October 2010.

Index

5-alpha-reductase type 2 deficiency, 47, 139

abdominal pain
  cyclical, 50–1, 146
adverse incidents
  use of reflective practice, 43, 131
amenorrhoea, 50–1, 146
amniocentesis
  detection of chromosome anomalies, 56, 156
  risk of miscarriage, 21, 88–9
amniotic fluid
  blood-stained, 59, 161–2
anabolic steroids
  effects on male fertility, 48, 141–2
androgen insensitivity syndrome, 47, 139
antibiotics
  contraceptive failure caused by, 55–6, 155
anti-c antibodies
  management in pregnancy, 51–2, 147–8
anticoagulant prophylaxis, 13, 75
anti-D antibodies
  management during pregnancy, 50, 145
anti-D immunoglobulin for rhesus D prophylaxis, 10, 68–9
anti-D prophylaxis
  indications for, 47–8, 139
antidepressants
  antenatal and postnatal use, 23, 92–3
antihypertensive agents, 15, 58, 79, 159
anti-La antibodies, 11, 71–2
antiphospholipid syndrome, 23, 93–4
anti-Ro antibodies, 11, 71–2
appraisal meetings, 42, 129–30
appraisal process, 16, 80–1
array comparative genomic hybridization (CGH), 56, 156
aspirin treatment, 11, 70–1
assessment methods, 16, 80–1
assessment tools, 10, 69
assisted reproduction
  bilateral hydrosalpinges, 9–10, 68
asthma

appropriate postpartum antihypertensive, 58, 159
deterioration in pregnancy, 42, 128
exacerbations during pregnancy, 33, 111–12
medication during labour and postpartum, 32, 110–11
autoimmune disease, 11, 41, 71–2, 127
autonomic dysreflexia
  risk in pregnant women with SCI, 52, 148–9
azoospermia
  and anabolic steroids, 48, 141–2
  cause in male with cystic fibrosis, 46, 136
  causes, 48, 141–2

bacterial sepsis following pregnancy, 14, 15, 30, 76, 78, 107–8
  causative organisms, 35, 115
  symptoms, 35, 115
bacterial sepsis in pregnancy
  maternal mortality rate, 15–16, 79–80
  risk of maternal mortality, 34, 114
bipolar disorder
  risk of postpartum psychosis, 25, 97
bleeding disorders, 24, 94–5
blood tests
  liver function tests, 18, 84
blood transfusion
  blood type for pregnant women, 41, 127–8
  management during pregnancy, 41, 127–8
BRCA mutations
  ovarian and breast cancer risks, 26, 99
breech presentation
  external cephalic version (ECV), 50, 144
  rate of spontaneous version, 50, 144

caesarean section, 12, 73
  nerve injury associated with, 33, 112
  risk of massive obstetric haemorrhage, 48, 140
cardiotocography, 59, 162

163

Index

cardiovascular system
  changes in pregnancy, 17, 82–3
cervical cerclage, 12, 73
  indications for, 40, 126
cervical cytopathology
  management, 35, 116
cervical intraepithelial neoplasia (CIN), 10, 69–70
  incomplete excision, 19–20, 25, 86, 98
cervical smear
  frequency after CIN excision, 25, 98
  frequency for HIV-positive patient, 22, 92
cervix
  premalignant disease, 55, 154
  transformation zone, 55, 154
chickenpox
  exposure during pregnancy, 23, 31, 53, 94, 109, 150
Chlamydia trachomatis
  neonatal infections, 43, 130
Chlamydia treatment, 12, 72–3
chorioamnionitis
  diagnosis, 59, 162
chromosome anomalies
  detection of, 56, 156
chronic kidney disease
  risk of pre-eclampsia, 37, 119
coagulation system
  changes in pregnancy, 17, 82–3
congenital adrenal hyperplasia, 47, 139
congenital bilateral absence of the vas deferens (CBAVD), 46, 136
contraception
  and treatment for *Chlamydia*, 12, 72–3
  drug interactions with hormonal contraception, 55–6, 155
  emergency, 12, 28, 72–3, 103–4
  levonorgestrel-releasing intrauterine system, 44, 133
  long-term, 44, 133
  missed pill recommendations, 9, 67
  time interval after delivery, 44, 133
  VTE risk with combined oral contraceptives, 46, 137
contraceptives
  cervical cap with spermicide, 46, 136
  medical eligibility classification, 30, 106–7
cyclical abdominal pain, 50–1, 146
cystic fibrosis
  azoospermia in male partner, 46, 136–7
  pattern of inheritance, 29, 36–7, 104
cytomegalovirus (CMV) infection
  risk of vertical transmission, 52, 149

delivery
  indications for operative delivery, 53, 150–1
depression
  antidepressant use in pregnancy, 23, 92–3
  risk of postpartum psychosis, 25, 97
dermatographia artefacta, 52–3, 149–50
diabetes
  risk factors, 11, 70–1
  screening, 11, 70–1
  See also gestational diabetes
drug interactions with hormonal contraception, 55–6, 155

early fetal demise management, 26, 100
early-onset neonatal group B streptococcal disease
  prevention of, 45, 48, 49, 53, 134, 140, 143–4, 150
eclampsia, 41, 127
ectopic pregnancy, 17–18, 47–8, 83–4, 139
emergency contraception, 9, 12, 67, 72–83
  drug combinations, 28, 103–4
endometrial polyps
  diagnosis, 13, 74–5
enhanced recovery in gynaecology, 16, 81
epilepsy
  management during pregnancy, 42, 128–9
  risk of peripartum seizures, 42, 128–9
external cephalic version (ECV), 50, 144

face presentation
  engaging diameter, 27–8, 102
  head delivery, 28, 103
faecal incontinence, 13, 75–6
faecal urgency
  following perineal tear, 37–8, 120–1
female genital mutilation (FGM), 9, 67–8
femoral nerve
  injury associated with hysterectomy, 11–12, 14, 31, 57, 72, 76–7, 108–9, 158–9
fertility assessment, 10–11, 70
fetal bleeding, 59, 161–2
fetal heart pattern
  sinusoidal trace, 59, 161–2
fetal hydrops. *See* hydrops fetalis
fetal infections
  prenatal diagnosis and management, 52, 149
fetal loss
  listeriosis, 39, 123
fetal mortality rate
  in non-immune hydrops fetalis, 42, 129
fetal movements
  reduced, 19, 47, 85–6, 138
fetomaternal haemorrhage (FMH), 10, 68–9
fetus
  congenital heart block risk, 29, 105
  heart block related to autoimmune disease, 11, 41, 71–2, 127
  shoulder dystocia, 48, 141
  small for gestational age, 41, 126
fibroids, 11–12, 31, 40, 72, 108–9, 125–6
  uterine artery embolization (UAE), 22, 91

genetic testing
  following third miscarriage, 18, 84
  recurrent miscarriage, 27, 101
gestational diabetes, 11, 70–1
  diagnostic criteria, 56, 156–7
gestational trophoblastic disease, 28, 102–3
  follow-up, 33, 113
  partial moles, 43–4, 132
gestational trophoblastic neoplasia (GTN)
  management, 33, 113
group A streptococcal (GAS) disease
  necrotizing fasciitis, 58–9, 160–1
  puerperal sepsis, 58–9, 159–61
group B streptococcal (GBS) disease
  prevention of early-onset neonatal infection, 48, 49, 140, 143–4

164

haematological changes during pregnancy, 25, 96–7
haemolytic disease of the newborn, 51–2, 147–8
head delivery
 in a face presentation, 28, 103
HELLP syndrome, 41, 127
heparin
 venous thrombosis prophylaxis, 12–13, 74
history-taking assessment, 10, 69
HIV infection in pregnancy
 effectiveness of HAART, 32, 111
 labour and delivery, 58, 160
 management, 11, 58, 71, 160
 management of labour, 57, 157–8
 reduction of mother to child transmission, 32, 111
 risk of vertical transmission, 39–40, 124
HIV-positive patient
 frequency of cervical smears, 22, 92
human papilloma virus (HPV)
 type responsible for vaginal disease, 32, 110
hydrops fetalis, 14, 77
hydrops fetalis (non-immune)
 fetal mortality rate, 42, 129
hydrosalpinges, 9–10, 68
hyperandrogenism
 differential diagnosis, 56, 155–6
hypertension
 postpartum, 15, 79
hypertension in pregnancy, 22, 41, 90–1, 127
 See also pre-eclampsia
hypogonadotropic hypogonadism in males, 48, 141–2
hysterectomy, 10, 40, 69–70, 125–6
 nerve injury associated with, 11–12, 14, 31, 51, 57, 72, 76–7, 108–9, 146–7, 158–9
 vaginal vault prolapse, 59, 161
hysteroscopes, 15, 78–9
hysteroscopy
 pain control, 20, 88
 reducing procedure-related pain, 40, 124–5
 uterine perforation, 21, 89–90

ilioinguinal nerve
 injury associated with hysterectomy, 51, 146–7
imperforate hymen, 50–1, 146
induction of labour, 19, 85–6
infanticide, 25, 97
infections
 risk of vertical transmission, 52, 149
infertility
 assessment of male infertility, 48, 141–2
 azoospermia in male with cystic fibrosis, 46, 136
 bilateral hydrosalpinges, 9–10, 68
 congenital bilateral absence of the vas deferens (CBAVD), 46, 136
 effects of male anabolic steroid use, 48, 141–2
 male hypogonadotropic hypogonadism, 48, 141–2
 treatments, 10–11, 70
 unexplained, 10–11, 70
inherited bleeding disorders, 24, 94–5

intrapartum pyrexia
 risk of early-onset neonatal group B streptococcal disease, 45, 134
itching in pregnancy, 52–3, 149–50
IVF treatment, 10–11, 70
 bilateral hydrosalpinges, 9–10, 68

karyotyping, 18, 84

labour
 active management of third stage, 53–4, 151
 continuous support during, 24, 96
 diagnosis of delay in first stage, 38, 121–2
 indications for operative delivery, 53, 150–1
 induced, 19, 85–6
 management of delay in first stage, 38, 121–2
 prolonged third stage, 47, 138
laparoscopic surgery
 ureteric injury associated with, 34–5, 115
laparoscopy
 avoiding entry-related injuries, 31, 43, 109–10, 131–2
 intra-abdominal pressure, 21, 43, 89, 131–2
levonorgestrel-releasing intrauterine contraceptive system, 44, 133
lidocaine
 dosage, 16, 80
 toxicity symptoms, 16, 80
listeriosis
 and preterm fetal loss, 39, 123
liver function tests, 18, 84
local anaesthetic
 lidocaine dosage, 16, 80
low-molecular-weight heparin (LMWH), 12–13, 74

magnesium toxicity
 signs of, 45–6, 135–6
malaria in pregnancy, 35–6, 116–17
male infertility
 assessment of, 48, 141–2
 effects of anabolic steroids, 48, 141–2
malpresentation, 28, 103
massive obstetric haemorrhage
 risk with placenta praevia, 48, 140
maternal morbidity
 risk factors, 12, 73–4
maternal mortality
 direct and indirect causes, 25, 97–8
 impact of obesity, 49, 142–3
 postpartum psychosis, 25, 97
 rate in severe sepsis, 15–16, 79–80
 risk factors, 12, 73–4
 risk in bacterial sepsis, 34, 114
 risk in septic shock, 34, 114
 sepsis mortality risk factors, 17, 83
 suicide, 25, 97
Mayer–Rokitansky–Küster–Hauser (MRKH) syndrome, 47, 139
McRoberts' manoeuvre
 teaching, 48, 141
membrane rupture. *See* rupture of membranes
mifepristone dosage, 26, 100
mini-CEX (mini clinical evaluation exercise), 10, 69

Index

miscarriage
  antiphospholipid syndrome, 23, 93–4
  cause of recurrent miscarriage, 23, 93–4
  causes of first-trimester miscarriage, 44, 133
  diagnosis in early pregnancy, 17–18, 83–4
  genetic testing, 18, 27, 84, 101
  incomplete, 27, 101
  indications for anti-D prophylaxis, 47–8, 139
  investigating recurrent first-trimester miscarriages, 45, 134–5
  management of future pregnancy, 46–7, 137
  prevention of recurrent unexplained miscarriage, 49, 142
  recurrent, 26–7, 36, 100, 101, 118
  risk following three consecutive miscarriages, 36, 118
  risk of further miscarriages, 49, 142
  risk with amniocentesis, 21, 88–9
misoprostol dosage, 26, 100
missed pill recommendations, 9, 67
molar pregnancy, 28, 102–3
  chromosomal composition of partial moles, 43–4, 132
monochorionic twin pregnancy, 20, 87
multiparous women
  reducing the risk of postpartum haemorrhage, 53–4, 151
myasthenia gravis
  drugs to avoid in pregnancy, 39, 123–4

necrotizing fasciitis
  diagnosis and management, 58–9, 160–1
neonatal chlamydial infections, 43, 130
neonatal conjunctivitis
  causative organisms, 43, 130
neonatal resuscitation training, 56–7, 157
neonatal varicella infection, 44–5, 133–4
nerve injury
  associated with caesarean section, 33, 112
  associated with hysterectomy, 11–12, 14, 31, 51, 57, 72, 76–7, 108–9, 146–7, 158–9
  associated with sacrospinous fixation, 36, 117
  indications of obturator nerve injury, 38–9, 122
nocturia
  management options, 38, 121
  treatment for frail older patients, 51, 147

obesity
  and polycystic ovarian syndrome, 51, 146
  impact on pregnant women, 49, 142–3
  maternal sepsis mortality risk, 17, 83
  risk of maternal morbidity and mortality, 12, 73–4
obstetric cholestasis
  itching associated with, 52–3, 149–50
obturator nerve injury
  motor findings, 38–9, 122
occipito-posterior presentation, 28, 103
oral contraceptive pill
  contraindications, 30, 106–7
oral glucose tolerance test (OGTT), 56, 156–7
outpatient diagnostic hysteroscopy
  pain control, 20, 88
ovarian cancer
  five-year survival, 37, 119–20
  staging, 37, 119–20
ovarian cancer risk
  and *BRCA* mutations, 26, 99
  lifetime risk in the general population, 27, 101
ovarian cysts
  in postmenopausal women, 40, 125
  in premenopausal women, 20, 86–7
  management, 29, 104–5
  management of simple small cysts, 54–5, 153
  surgical management, 40, 125
ovarian masses
  management, 29, 30, 104, 106
ovarian torsion
  diagnosis and management, 30, 107
ovarian tumour markers, 30, 106
overactive bladder, 21, 90
  management options, 38, 121
  treatment, 23, 93
  treatment for frail older patients, 51, 147

pain
  diagnosis of pudendal neuralgia, 54, 153
partial moles
  chromosomal composition, 43–4, 132
parvovirus infection in pregnancy, 14, 77
pelvic fracture
  pregnant patient, 31, 108
perineal tears, 13, 22, 75–6, 91–2
  classification, 43, 130–1
  faecal urgency following, 37–8, 120–1
  outcome following primary repair, 37–8, 120–1
periods
  infrequent, 51, 146
persistent trophoblast, 18–19, 85
personal development plan, 42, 129–30
placenta
  prolonged third stage of labour, 47, 138
placenta praevia
  risk of massive obstetric haemorrhage, 48, 140
placental abruption
  risk in a subsequent pregnancy, 24, 95–6
polycystic ovary syndrome, 51, 146
  differential diagnosis, 56, 155–6
polymorphic eruption of pregnancy, 26, 99–100
POPQ scoring system
  vaginal vault, 59, 161
postmenopausal vulval itching, 44, 132
postnatal fever and rigor, 58–9, 159–61
postpartum depression, 25, 97
postpartum haemorrhage
  reducing the risk of, 53–4, 151
postpartum hypertension, 15, 79
  antihypertensive for asthmatic patient, 58, 159
postpartum psychosis
  risk factors, 25, 97
pre-conception counselling
  antidepressant use in pregnancy, 23, 92–3
  risk of postpartum psychosis, 25, 97
pre-eclampsia
  management, 37, 120

risk factors, 37, 119
risk in subsequent pregnancies, 41, 49, 127, 143
risk of recurrence, 22, 90–1
signs of magnesium toxicity, 45–6, 135–6
presenting diameter, 28, 103
professional development needs
　use of reflective practice, 43, 131
progestogens
　VTE risk in combined oral contraceptives, 46, 137
pruritis in pregnancy, 26, 52–3, 99–100, 149–50
pudendal nerve
　injury associated with sacrospinous fixation, 36, 117
　three branches, 55, 154–5
pudendal nerve block, 55, 154–5
pudendal neuralgia
　diagnosis, 54, 153
puerperal sepsis, 14, 76
　diagnosis and management, 58, 159–60
　group A streptococcal (GAS) disease, 58–9, 160–1

recurrent urinary tract infections (UTIs), 50, 145
reduced fetal movements, 19, 47, 85–6, 138
reflective practice, 43, 131
relative risk
　explanation of, 54, 152
resuscitation training, 56–7, 157
retained products of conception
　risks associated with surgical evacuation, 45, 135
rhesus D prophylaxis, 10, 68–9
risk
　explanation of relative risk, 54, 152
　ways to explain, 20, 87–8
rupture of membranes
　preterm pre-labour rupture, 49, 59, 143–4, 162

sacrospinous fixation
　nerve injury associated with, 36, 117
salpingectomy, 18–19, 85
salpingostomy, 18–19, 85
sepsis
　diagnosis and management, 58, 159–60
　group A streptococcal (GAS) disease, 58–9, 160–1
　group A streptococcal (GAS) puerperal sepsis, 58, 159–60
　risk factors for maternal mortality, 17, 83
septic shock, 30, 107–8
　risk of maternal mortality, 34, 114
severe maternal sepsis, 15, 30, 78, 107–8
　mortality rate, 15–16, 79–80
　risk factors, 12, 73–4
shoulder dystocia, 14–15, 48, 77–8, 141
sickle cell disease
　management in pregnancy, 33, 112–13
　pattern of inheritance, 33, 112–13
sickle cell trait
　pattern of inheritance, 33, 112–13
simple ovarian cyst
　management, 29, 104–5
simulation training, 14–15, 77–8

Sjögren's syndrome antibodies, 11, 71–2
skills development
　simulation training, 14–15, 77–8
skin conditions in pregnancy, 26, 52–3, 99–100, 149–50
slapped cheek syndrome in pregnancy, 14, 77
spinal cord injury (SCI)
　pregnancy care plan, 52, 148–9
　risks associated with pregnancy, 52, 148–9
spontaneous vaginal delivery
　influential factors, 24, 96
statistical tests, 35, 115–16
suicide (maternal), 25, 97
surgery
　instruments causing uterine perforation, 32, 110
　nerve injury associated with, 11–12, 14, 31, 36, 51, 57, 72, 76–7, 108–9, 117, 146–7, 158–9
　sites of uterine perforation, 34, 114
　ureteric injury associated with, 34–5, 115
　WHO surgical sign out, 16–17, 81–2
suture absorption
　time taken, 55, 154
suture materials
　appropriate choice of, 55, 154
Swyer's syndrome, 47, 139
systemic lupus erythematosus (SLE)
　in pregnancy, 11, 41, 71–2, 127
　maternal and fetal complications, 29, 105

teaching methods
　simulation training, 14–15, 77–8
teratogenic drugs, 39, 123–4
testosterone
　raised serum levels in women, 56, 155–6
thalassaemia
　cardiac iron overload, 36, 117–18
　management in pregnancy, 29, 36, 105–6, 117–18
thrombophilia screening, 25, 39, 96–7, 122–3
transformation zone of the cervix, 55, 154
truncus arteriosus
　detection of cause, 56, 156
tubal pregnancy, 18–19, 85
tumour markers
　ovarian tumours, 30, 106
twins
　management of delivery, 57, 158
　monochorionic twin pregnancy, 20, 50, 87, 144–5
　prognosis following single-twin death, 50, 144–5

umbilical artery Doppler, 41, 126
unexplained infertility, 10–11, 70
ureters
　injury associated with surgery, 34–5, 115
urinary frequency
　management options, 38, 121
urinary incontinence, 21, 90
　treatment for frail older patients, 51, 147
urinary tract infection (UTI)
　recurrent infections, 50, 145
urinary urgency
　management options, 38, 121
　treatment for frail older patients, 51, 147

Index

uterine artery embolization (UAE), 22, 91
uterine inversion, 26, 98–9
uterine perforation
  during hysteroscopy, 21, 89–90
  instruments causing, 32, 110
  most common sites, 34, 114
  procedures associated with risk of, 54, 152
  risk in postpartum procedures, 45, 135
utero-vaginal prolapse, 50, 145

vagina
  congenital abnormalities, 47, 139
vaginal carcinoma
  HPV type responsible, 32, 110
vaginal delivery
  influential factors in spontaneous delivery, 24, 96
vaginal vault cytology, 10, 40, 69–70, 125–6
vaginal vault on POPQ scoring system, 59, 161
vaginal vault prolapse, 59, 161
  frail elderly patient, 38, 122
  indications for colpocleisis, 38, 122

varicella-zoster virus
  infection in pregnancy, 23, 31, 44–5, 94, 109, 133–4
vasa praevia, 59, 161–2
  diagnosis and management, 34, 113–14
venous thromboembolism (VTE)
  incidence in pregnancy and the puerperium, 24, 95
  prophylaxis, 12–13, 74, 75
  risk factors, 13, 75
  risk in pregnancy, 17, 82–3
  risk in pregnant patients with thalassaemia, 29, 105–6
  risk of heritable thrombophilia, 39, 122–3
  risk with combined oral contraceptives, 46, 137
  thrombophilia screen, 39, 122–3
viral rash in pregnancy, 14, 77
von Willebrand's disease, 24, 94–5
vulva
  lesion treatment, 22–3, 92
  pain and itching, 27, 101–2
  postmenopausal itching, 44, 132
vulval dermatitis, 27, 101–2